SACRED MEDICINE

MYSTICAL PRACTICES FOR ECSTATIC LIVING

JEN PICENO

FEATURING: ASHERAH ALLEN, DR. JOSIE BEUG , SUSAN CONNOR, ALIESHA DAVIS, DARLENE DE LA PLATA, EIRIKAH DELAUNAY, AMBER DOBKINS, MELISSA JOLLY GRAVES, DR. STEPHANIE RAE GRENIER, KATY JO HOLTON, JAMES KEALIIPIILANI KAWAINUI, MORRIGHAN LYNNE, LAURA MAZZOTTA, CAROLYN MCGEE, KELLY MYERSON, LYNN OLIVARI, DOUGLAS RARDEN, DARBY RYON, SARAH SPARKS, LULU TREVENA, MELANIE WELLER, VICTORIA WELSH, ATLANTIS WOLF, CHELSEA LEE WOUDSTRA

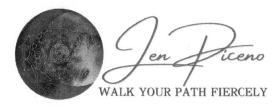

WALK YOUR PATH FIERCELY

Grab your free Abundance for Unlimited Possibilities audio meditation at
https://www.JenPiceno.com/Resources

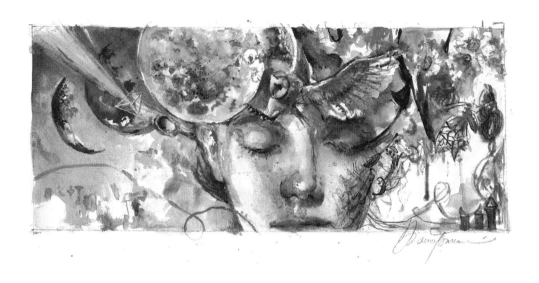

Holding a master's degree in Fine Arts from the prestigious Romanian University of Art and Design in Cluj-Napoca, Diana has been engaging with the art community since 1995 showcasing her work in over a hundred international group exhibitions and eight solo art shows. Diana is often invited to judge and jury art shows and to speak on behalf of the working artist on open panels, such as The Mayor's Office of Cultural Affairs, and at The Contemporary Museum in Atlanta, Georgia. Between 1995 and 2021 Diana won an array of awards locally as well as on an international level. Her artworks have been showcased in art magazines, billboards, and acquired by corporations to be displayed in public spaces. Diana is the demonstration chair for Georgia Watercolor Society and the former IWS USA branch president of the International Watercolor Society. Diana also teaches painting classes for adults in the Atlanta area and at art centers within the US and abroad. Her teaching approach focuses on fast, free-flowing painting release, and creative un-blockage.

www.ArtByDianaToma.com

YOU ARE THE MEDICINE

"Cure yourself with the light of the sun and the rays of the moon.

With the sound of the river and the waterfall.

With the swaying of the sea and the fluttering of birds.

Heal yourself, with the mint and mint leaves,

with neem and eucalyptus.

Sweeten yourself with lavender,

rosemary, and chamomile.

Hug yourself with the cocoa bean and a touch of cinnamon.

Put love in tea instead of sugar and take it looking at the stars.

Heal yourself, with the kisses that the wind gives you

and the hugs of the rain.

Get strong with bare feet on the ground and

with everything that is born from it.

Get smarter every day by listening to your intuition,

looking at the world with the eye of your forehead.

Jump, dance, sing, so that you live happier.

Heal yourself, with beautiful love,

and always remember… you are the medicine."

~Maria Sabina
Mexican Curandera (healer) and Poet.

SACRED MEDICINE
INTENTION STATEMENT

May we embody the power of divine love, magic, wisdom, and sacredness to reawaken the strength of our unique spiritual gifts and use them for the highest good.

May we confidently inspire, ignite, and activate change in our lives and the lives of others.

May we honor and trust this mystical path, sharing our gifts wisely, passionately, fiercely, and intentionally with sacred purpose.

May this tribe of talented medicine men and women be all that they came here to be, and more for all who read this book.

May you, and all of our readers, evolve into the next highest version of yourself and beyond.

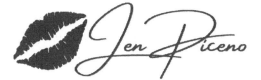

DEDICATION

My deepest gratitude to all the coaches, healers, teachers, and mystics who have impacted my life and empowered this path of transformation. I am forever grateful.

To the people who have challenged, hurt, or betrayed me, you unknowingly gifted me opportunities to grow through my pain and suffering. Thank you for pushing me to the edge—it's where I learned how to spread my wings and fly upon the air of transformation.

To our courageous authors, thank you for sharing your SACRED MEDICINE with the world. I feel your power, know your integrity, trust your wisdom, and am deeply honored to have you in my tribe.

SPECIAL NOTE TO THE READER

Dear sweet soul,

Envision yourself encircled by twenty-five powerful medicine people who gathered to witness your healing, celebrate your magic, and honor your wisdom.

They were wounded once, long ago, but vowed to transform their pain into "sacred medicine" to restore health, awaken magic, and bring light into areas of darkness. What once poisoned their spirit no longer exists. It has been blended and ground into powerful medicine with pure intentions, love, and lessons learned. It's being offered to you now in a handmade cup blessed by the elders.

The deep sound of the drum pulses in sync with your heartbeat, and it brings your attention inward. The rattle shimmers and shakes over your body to purify your mind, body, and spirit. It releases suppressed emotions, and your body dissolves all tension, along with any negative or stagnant energy.

Smoke billows up toward the starlit sky with the scent of sage as it blesses the land you stand on. As the earth kisses the soles of your feet, you connect with her. This is your welcoming home.

With your next inhale, sacredness fills every fiber of your being.

In celebration, we drum, dance, and chant in your honor for this transformative spiritual awakening. It's a tribute to your self-realization and the invitation to reclaim personal power, magic, and mystery.

As you journey through these pages, do so with an open heart so you can receive the beauty waiting for you. Skip from chapter to chapter and read whatever calls your attention.

Trust the process; you're being led to exactly where you need to go.

Let the journey begin.

TABLE OF CONTENTS

INTRODUCTION

My voice cracked as I spoke to myself, "I can't keep doing this." My eyes burned as the tears poured out in a steady stream. The taste of salt rolled over my lips, and my cheeks stained from watery emotions rolling down my face. Every muscle tightened as if holding on for dear life and dying all at the same time. The intensity of my feelings was uncharted territory. I was lost.

I felt defeated, empty, and hopeless with no sense of clarity other than something had to change. I struggled to move through the day.

My physical body was exhausted, and emotionally I had nothing left to give. I was in love, yet the pains of the past haunted my heart. I cried, screamed, and moaned, feeling all the grief and disappointment of how I lost myself somewhere along the way.

Then, magically an opportunity showed up. I didn't have enough money for this transformational offer that teased my spirit and left me aching inside.

In the depth of uncertainty, I walked outside to get some fresh air. A crow swooped down "caw, caw," announcing his magical presence. I walked to the mailbox, touching the trees along the way and feeling the chill of the earth beneath my bare feet as the dew anointed my soles with each step forward.

Abracadabra! My emotions calmed as if someone had waved a magic wand over my head. I snatched the mail from the mailbox, and there was a royalty check from a TV show I had been on years long ago. Get this! It was exactly enough to cover the priestess training. It was a cosmic wink with a gift from the divine.

I decided to step onto this path of self-discovery to rid myself of this suffering.

I entered the program to heal myself, find clarity, understanding, and purpose. I sought after answers but emerged as "KatFyre," Priestess, activator of change and transformation. I received clear visions and integrated power more generous than I could have ever imagined.

I discovered the power of the sacred medicine I carry in my unique medicine bag as a priestess, medicine woman, and practitioner of the sacred arts.

I harnessed divine feminine power and infused it with the strength offered by the inner masculine in sacred marriage of self. The holy feminine emerged with the desire to create, receive pleasure, and manifest desires into form.

This new energy rippled through me, and I felt fully supported as an innovative leader instead of feeling bullied or hidden away. The masculine became my protector, offering support and paving the way for the creations longing to be birthed through me. It solved the internal conflict that had been self-sabotaging me for decades. I found inner peace, and it changed everything.

Intuition, wisdom, and life force energy stirred and brought me back to life. Powerful inner wisdom lead me forward with a supercharged presence and magnetism bigger and bolder than I ever had as a professional dancer.

I moved fast! Healing from the inside out, I was revitalized back into health and happiness. Intentions were fueled with purpose, and I vowed to ascend to the highest heights my soul could reach while leading others to do the same.

Through ceremony, ritual, and foundational spiritual practices, I discovered pleasure in simple everyday moments. I found a deep appreciation for all things and began living in everyday ceremony. I celebrate life with pure ecstatic joy because I deserve it, and so do you.

It's juicy and delicious, and I want it to be accessible to everyone ready to receive the vibrant life force energy, love, and abundance available.

I was lead to share SACRED MEDICINE with you through visions of gathering medicine men and women together to share their stories, ceremonies, rituals, and practices to inspire, encourage, and lead you into life-changing magnificence.

Step into the magical world of self-discovery, deep healing, accentuated pleasure, heightened intuition, and the liberating feeling of ecstatic living.

You're here with great purpose. It's your turn! Go ahead, start claiming the sweet nectar of life.

Flip through these pages to receive the medicine we collectively share. Your life experiences hold power, wisdom, and potent medicine.

It's time to handcraft your unique magical potion, soul-expanding medicine, and healing salve by trusting the process and leaping into happiness.

You're a divine being with the power to transform everything that has caused you harm, struggle, heartache, or disappointment.

The transformation begins now.

CHAPTER 1
LIFE-FORCE ENERGY ACTIVATION

IGNITING WEALTH CONSCIOUSNESS AND DIVINE TRUTH

Jen Piceno, Priestess ORDM, Wealth Consciousness Coach

"She loved the mystery so much, she became one."

MY STORY

My body twitched with intense vibration. Something ignited within me with intense purpose. A blast of energy tingled up my spine. Woosh! Whole-body chills, then another wave of excessive heat. She activated something, and I couldn't quite grasp what was happening. It was mystical and magical–completely beyond logical understanding.

She pulled me onto the stage, and without hesitation, I eagerly followed. I was in a Deja Vu trance-like state, knowing everything that was about to happen and understanding none of it all at the same time.

She stood firmly grounded with her feet planted underneath her round hips while a soft smile danced upon her lips. I felt the warmth of her breath as she inched in face-to-face, grasping my hands into hers. "Let's get started." My heartbeat accelerated in anticipation, yet I was calm—a deep knowing that life was about to change anchored me into the experience.

The small, sturdy South African woman cupped her hands around my face and blew into the crown of my head, owning her divine power and attuning me to mine. This experience was an invitation to the bigger vision and called me to action.

Tap-tap-tap, her hand thumped my upper chest then firmly swept over my shoulders from one to the other. Tension vanished, my ears tingled, and my chest beaded with sweat. She spoke softly with divine authority, "make a sound, any sound." Something was happening. My vision was crystal clear, and everything brilliantly vibrant. Her voice angelically washed over me "go on dear, make a sound, any sound." It was weird, but I followed her instructions.

I stared back in wonder, trying to find my voice. My throat tingled with a sparkling vibration. The sound was trying to come, but first, a burst of laughter, then tears of joy shot out of my eyes. The laughter was pure divine happiness, and I couldn't stop even if I wanted to—it was magical and euphoric. The sounds were coming in just as she had instructed. "Go on, dear," she encouraged.

Shivers and tiny twitches vibrated up and down my spine. My eyes widened, and my tongue began to move at warp speed. Vitality pumped through my blood and bones as I spoke the "original language," a brilliant language of light. Radiance poured through me as if welcoming me home to myself with a surge of life-force energy. It was familiar but mysterious all at the same time.

I don't know how my mouth kept up speaking so rapidly in this foreign tongue. The connection was instant. My body merged with heaven and earth while my soul expressed itself with the vibration of love, light, frequency, and sound.

Supercharged energy and aliveness led to ecstatic emotion rushing through me like a tidal wave. More divine laughter bubbled up while tears of joy flowed like sacred water. I wondered how any of this was possible and then instantaneously had the deep knowledge to *simply receive*. So, I did. I chose to soak it all up.

The heat built more robust and potent from the inside out as my body filled with golden light. The woman gazed into my eyes. The warmth of her hands melted into mine, "you are complete."

Those words vibrated through me with firm confirmation: *You are complete.*

It was as if I reinvented myself. There was an incredibly familiar adornment towards the woman standing before me. She was ancient and sacred. I knew her, yet I didn't. The sense of mystery was seductive and divine all the same time. My body needed time to integrate and understand the new me as my curiosities ran with wild abandon. Something had unlocked, and I was free.

After all of the excitement, I drove home feeling larger than life with a flawless spiritual high. Then it sunk in; what now? There were no further explanations of what happened—zero information on harnessing the power sourcing through me. I needed answers. The family said, "it's in the Bible, so it's good, it's a gift, right?" That's it! At seventeen-ish years old, that was a lot of energetic power to embrace without understanding what to do with it. So, I hid it away while the divine energy taught me everything I needed to know.

I spoke non-stop in private, cultivating the energy, feeling the vibration, and understanding its authentic meaning. It would "turn on" whenever something needed to be known or expressed. At times it annoyed the shit out of me! The wildly eclectic sounds would stream in as tribal, ancient, indigenous, and even alien-like at times. Thousands of tones and sounds came through me, then symbols, drawings, chants, and songs. I claimed and embodied this magic as my uniqueness while still hiding it away.

Fast forward to later in life, utterly heartbroken by my boyfriend (now husband). He was the bridge that brought hiding my secret to a sudden stop. Marching outside, I slammed the door behind me, tears streaming. Intense sounds came roaring from the pit of my belly—no controlling it. Ancient wisdom through fierce soul language flowed through me. A language from the beginning of time passionately flew out of my mouth with explosive power and strength. I understood everything through my senses. The meaning and translation were experienced through me and deeply understood.

I was being schooled, guided, and taught through divine wisdom. *This is happening for you. Claim the lessons and grow from the experience. You have everything you need to break ancestral patterns, dissolve fears and challenges, and to move through everything with purpose. Harness this wisdom with divine power and teach others to do the same.*

Then, he came bolting out the door bewildered by the sound which led him back to me. Surprisingly, he listened attentively with adornment in his eyes, his body softened, and he gently reached to embrace me as if he understood everything I was experiencing. I melted in his arms, feeling seen and held differently than ever before by anyone. I officially ended hiding the gifts.

The heaviness lifted as I savored pure self-acceptance accompanied by an overflow of happiness. Deep love blasted through me with the remembrance of lifetimes we've shared. I don't remember what the fight was about, but I'll forever remember how he scooped me up into his warm embrace while I experienced the sacred connection that crossed all time and space in my heart.

Deep-rooted knowing expanded me on all levels:

He chose to be in this lifetime with you for the grander vision of your mission. You will grow through each challenge. He will push you to your limits, and you will do the same for him. Together, you'll inspire growth, remembering who you are at more profound levels of existence. Each struggle and act of forgiveness offers loving celebration, expansion, and soulful evolution. The human experience shares pain and pleasure so that you'll rise and fly to new heights, heights beyond the human mind's comprehension. Delight in the whole experience and learn all that you can. Everything is happening for your ascension. It's part of the divine plan.

The messages resonated so deeply and guided me to save our relationship even in the most challenging times in our marriage when I wanted nothing more than to let go. Our deep-seated connection has prevailed against all odds through multiple lifetimes.

Years later, during a time of spiritual growth, I traveled to participate in the Gathering of the Shamans. The rituals and ceremonies activated my spiritual gifts with new awareness. Deep understanding poured through as I channeled knowledge from my ancestors and spirit guides. They showed me flashbacks of previous lifetimes like a movie playing in my head, then overlapped my years of training in eastern and western practices. Everything I had sought after, I had been and done before. Something mysteriously shifted with persuasive self-realization. My frequency ramped up in the vortexes bringing me into a more extensive alignment with my spiritual center. I said yes to every soul-expanding adventure and soaked up Sedona's masculine and feminine energies at each vortex. I shifted with each encounter, absorbing the guidance to serve at a deeper level.

A few women learned of my abilities, "would you be willing to work with us." Visions came, and messages flowed almost instantly. My senses accentuated, it was different than ever before. I pulled anger, grief, and self-loathing out of them. Everything purged through my physical body. I distinctly felt everything, all the pain, emotion, intense anger, fear, and disappointment. And under it all, a deep sorrow tangled in the webs of unhealed grief from decades of defeat. The intensity increased, and I couldn't hold back what had to be expressed.

I'm a sacred vessel of communication in channeling divine messages. This time, the messages came with English translations. It came in fiercely with refined purpose and crystal-clear clarity to activate change and transformation.

I hadn't shared this hidden healing gem of mine in client sessions before, so I didn't know it came with these extraordinary healing translations. Most healers don't have the gift of translation while channeling light language. I've been entrusted as a medicine woman to activate change, ignite transformation, and enhance lives with this powerful sacred medicine drenched in wealth consciousness.

I never needed translations for myself, but others do so they can embrace complete mind-body-spirit healing and fully receive the abundance of change it offers. From that day forward, I understood the power of my potent gifts and have shared them with all clients and students on their healing journey.

I AM AN ACTIVATOR OF CHANGE AND TRANSFORMATION - THIS IS MY SACRED MEDICINE.

Divine inspiration led me back to the mountains. The sky filled with vibrant red and orange as the sun set behind me. My body tingled, willing to receive the next activation in sacred ceremony with high priestesses, healers, shamans, and lightworkers. I stepped into the center of a twelve-foot crystal grid. My body was tingling as crystalline energy traveled up through my feet. Spirit connected me deeper into the sacred mysteries. I plugged into the core of my divine essence. Swaying like the wind with a gentle ebb and flow from left to right like a pendulum, I felt sacred, worthy, and powerful.

A stunning high priestess stepped into the crystal grid. Her hands lovingly laid upon my shoulders with a blessing from the elders and spirit guides. Holy oil scented of rose swept over my forehead, "you're anointed." Spirals of smoke billowed around my feet, filling the air with sage as a Toltec shaman fanned the smoke to encircle my body. The scent took me on a journey, and drumming synced with my heartbeat, bringing me into profound self-awareness.

A ceremony of self-ingratiation to infuse the divine masculine and feminine energies began with a blending of mystical opposites, becoming one in the "sacred marriage of self."

Emotions swirled through me, stimulating my spiritual, physical, emotional, and mental bodies. Then, springing into divine action, I claimed all the pieces of myself and released the need to be one or the other. Nothing was missing. I was whole. Divine wisdom flowed.

"This is the source of manifesting greatness. No longer will you work as half of yourself. You're whole. There's no need to struggle to get what you desire. The masculine supports the feminine as she brings things to life in manifested form, birthing them into creation. This union offers the highest frequency with the wholeness of consciousness. Bringing your masculine and feminine together in balance for divine integration allows you to create from a place of wholeness. The need to overwork and over give will diminish. You will release fears and encounter abundance all around you. Move into purpose to influence others. Align and attune them with sacred wholeness, activate their spiritual clarity, and serve as you're called to do."

Poof! I surrendered the hustle and quit working at the expense of my highest potential. Suddenly I realized that I fought against myself most of my life. An inner conflict between my divine masculine and divine feminine held me back from receiving abundance.

Now, everything flows. I get more done in less time. I'm energetically complete and stay in the state of wealth consciousness (money, health, freedom, relationships, creativity, spirituality). Abundance flows to me. I don't chase it!

In wholeness, we become ever-expansive and blessed with divine compensation anchored back into our sacred birthright. Step onto the path of totality and into heavenly states of wealth consciousness. You deserve to cross the threshold to align with abundance in every area of life. It's a rich and soulful journey that breaks limitations and sets us on a path to personal and financial freedom.

With 30+ years of channeling the divine and a variety of sacred practices to pull from, I simplify and speed up the process for women eager to take action in solving life's most challenging problems so they can consciously claim the life they deserve.

Receive my "medicine" below for a Life-Force Activation into wealth consciousness for your highest potential.

Join my private Facebook community. It's an online space for sacred sisterhood, wealth consciousness, and spiritual growth. https://www.facebook.com/groups/jenpiceno

Follow me on for juicy heart-felt wisdom, magical inspiration, and beautiful offerings. You'll find quick links here: https://linktr.ee/jenpiceno

THE MEDICINE

Wealth consciousness is the full experience of all things in life that bring us into wholeness. Our physical health, financial wealth, relationship fulfillment, emotional wellbeing, creative expression, and spiritual awareness integrated into one life amplifies ecstatic living with the energetic frequency of wealth on all levels of our existence.

WEALTH CONSCIOUSNESS ACTIVATION

Visit www.JenPiceno.com/resources for a complimentary recording of this activation with light language and translation.

The following channeled light language message was translated to English. The intention is to activate change in your life to the deepest, most intimate level you are willing to receive.

The frequency works on all levels of existence to enhance personal transformation, life-force energy, deeper awareness, and integrative wealth consciousness (health, freedom, relationship, love, wealth, creativity, and spirituality)

Be prepared to receive this sacred medicine. It's available to all; some will resist, turning their head away. But you, you are ready. Raise your hand upon your heart and receive as you expand to the fullest potential you are willing to receive.

I know you've been hurt, lost, and suffered on this journey of yours. All the wounds had a grander purpose. You're now offered the liberated freedom to transform it all. Take what once poisoned your spirit and use it to heal yourself fully, completely calling all the pieces of yourself back home.

You're not broken. I know you've felt it at times. Bring yourself back together and allow the golden light to fuse the pieces back. Coming back into fullness, snapping together like puzzle pieces. Each piece comes back home into your physical body. Feel the power coming back. Feel the love, the divinity, and the strength you have received from each experience. Bring the wisdom into your heart space and claim the lessons now.

As the last piece snaps together, with the highest vibration of light, you're activated. Child, remember who you are. Know the medicine you carry. In your vulnerability, harness your strength. In fear of your darkness, see the illumination of your divine light.

Allow yourself to feel whatever it is you need to feel. This is a gift of our humaneness. It's time for you to realize your inner beauty and claim everything you want and desire: Magic, mystery, joy, love, peace, balance, and harmony; all of it. The abundance of all things lives inside you.

You're connected to all that is, connected both to heaven and earth. You are not separate. You are not alone. You are part of the grander vision, and it is time for you to remember. Remember your divine inheritance and gaze upon the divine blueprint to help you navigate forward.

Fear not. You're being led. You must trust the wisdom that comes through as life-force energy penetrates you, receive the activation. Receive it now as you're invited to be activated into divine transformation. You are restoring your vitality, courage, strength and restoring the love and trust within yourself.

Child, you're enough. You're more than enough. The time has come for you to know that as truth. Allow this transmission to be completed by sealing the energy. Say out loud:

I receive this activation of transformation; I claim it as mine as I harness my power with trust in myself.

Bringing that into your body. Shifting your belief system at a cellular level, allowing all this energy to integrate within your physical form, receiving, receiving, receiving embrace this now; it is for you.

Take a deep breath in, and release. Wiggle your fingers and toes and come back to this time and space.

Grab a journal and start writing as fast as you can, allowing anything and everything to flow through you. Trust the process.

Thank you for being here. Thank you for receiving this transformation, this activation—this divine love.

Receive my channeled light language abundance activation "Abundance for Unlimited Possibilities" at https://www.JenPiceno.com/resouces

Private coaching, group programs, and sacred experiences available at https://www.JenPiceno.com

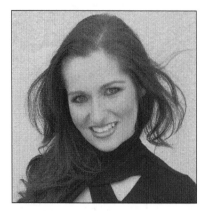

Jen Piceno, Priestess, ORDM, RTM, LMT, THP, is a business and spiritual coach specializing in wealth consciousness and life management. She is an expert energy medicine practitioner and medicine woman with 30+ years experience in the healing arts. Through personalized ceremony, ancestral healing, and channeling divine wisdom, she'll help you bust through restrictions so you can solidify your purpose and begin the transformation you've been craving in any area of your life.

Get ready to align with everything you were meant to be in ways you've never experienced before.

Jen is the CEO of Gypsy Moon Inc. and a lifetime student of spiritual practices attained from cultural wisdom worldwide.

She blends eastern and western modalities with light language, shamanic practices, and sacred ceremonies. Her work is infused with practices that activate the senses and alchemize challenges into purpose.

Jen is an ordained shamanic priestess in the lineage of StarrFire OrbWeaver, Anyaa McAndrew, and the creatrix, Nicole Christine. Walking the Priestess Path, she celebrates life in everyday ceremony and is committed to making a difference in the lives of others.

Jen is a double Reiki master and cross-trained in universal healing modalities. She's a scholar of the creative healing arts and an activator of change, transformation, and abundance.

Jen offers wealth consciousness coaching for personal and professional growth, shamanic healing, sacred ceremonies, personalized programs, spiritual development, and online training to encourage soul growth.

She is available in person and in her virtual sacred space. Visit: https://www.JenPiceno.com

Explore her free group on Facebook, where she shares her wisdom, strengthens sacred sisterhood, and inspires spiritual growth. Check out her videos on YouTube, or grab some freebies on her resource page.

Get access to all quick links here: https://linktr.ee/JenPiceno

CHAPTER 2

VAGUS NERVE COSMOLOGY

THE SPIRITUAL UNDERPINNINGS OF PHYSICAL DYSFUNCTION

Melanie Weller PT, MPT, OCS, CEEAA, ATC

"The greatest mistake in the treatment of disease is that there are physicians for the body and physicians for the soul, although the two cannot be separated."

-Plato

MY STORY

I felt giddy after finishing my December holiday stress management class. I got up from my meditation spot, the perch from which I taught. I was inspired to share my favorite image of my most loved anatomical structure ever on my social media channels.

Basking in the afterglow of increasing movement and decreasing pain in a group of people, the life I dreamt of, working a few hours per day from the Swiss Alps, felt closer than ever.

Treating people over the internet is so much more fun than treating patients in person. Class isn't the right word for what I am doing. What is it? Part teaching, part meditation, part energy healing. It's a show. A healing show! Act 1, Meditation. Act 2, Teaching, Act 3, Healing others through the ethers.

I laughed at myself. Performing was not in my repertoire of skills. A few years ago, using my physical therapy skills through the ethers was not in my repertoire, either.

I hadn't planned on talking so much about the ventricles of the brain. I did, as intended, teach the vagus nerve's structure and function. I taught how to treat it as a pinched nerve and did my own manual therapy intervention. I just did it from hundreds or thousands of miles away from these people. As I treated the first individual, the symptoms in the other participants dissipated, and quickly everyone was both objectively and subjectively improved.

I spent thirty years collecting professional credentials to validate my knowledge. Yet, I feel like I have known how to do remote energy healing for all eternity without any formal training.

I opened my Sobotta Anatomy book to snap a photo of the rendering and post it on social media. A compilation of MRI scans showed a three-dimensional rendering of the ventricles of the brain. This time, when I opened the book, I saw something very different.

Sharing my favorite anatomical structure was always a joy. I had shared this image in person with patients many times since I purchased Sobotta Anatomy to go along with a series of continuing education courses that referenced the images in this edition. I became obsessed with the ventricles after taking Craniosacral Osteopathic Technique from Michigan State University's College of Osteopathic Medicine. Dr. Philip Greenman, the head physician at the time, said that our cranial rhythms, the pulse of our cerebrospinal fluid pumping, lasted about 20 minutes after the time of death. This mind-blowing fact about my beloved ventricles left me in a state of wonder. I remembered the two questions they always evoked in me.

How much momentum must be in the system to make it last that long?

Was the ceasing of the cranial rhythmic impulse the actual time of death, the time when our souls leave our bodies?

The image of the ventricles reminded me of the propulsion section of the Enterprise from Star Trek or some kind of alien spaceship. To me, the ventricles were a propulsion system, even if, in conventional terms, their function was to make cerebrospinal fluid that cushioned, fed, and cleansed the central nervous system.

I always used lots of metaphors when explaining anatomy to patients. It was an easy way to communicate what was happening in their bodies. I always found value in hearing, metaphorically, what they felt was going on. My hands-on intervention and exercises would untangle the knot, wring out the full sponge, or remove the ice pick, even if the interventions seemed markedly similar. I intentionally designed treatment programs to treat these metaphors and reflected this language back to my patients. My patients called me "The Body Whisperer" because I could resolve situations quickly and easily when no one else could. Using metaphor was an integral part of my whispering skills.

Staring at the picture I had looked at a million times before, my heart skipped a beat, and goosebumps washed over my body.

My sweet ventricles look precisely like the symbol for Aries!

I had been in the throes of a proverbial mid-life crisis and was home doing this class because I had declared myself retired from physical therapy. I moved out of my office and stayed home to reimagine what my business could look like and create an online presence. It was also accurate to say the stress was so intense I blew up my thriving practice. My previously rock-solid marriage felt like it was on shaky ground. My blood pressure was high. I couldn't get rid of my foot pain. I had a professional lawsuit pending. The plaintiff was someone I considered a friend and the only person I treated for free.

My life was falling apart. Everything I thought was solid was coming undone. So I started studying astrology to understand why. One of my patients had an old friend who was now doing astrology. The connection came up very serendipitously, and it felt like confirmation that this was something I needed to pursue.

I naturally gravitated towards medical astrology. Each body part and system was "ruled" by a specific planet and its corresponding constellation. So I searched online for a list of anatomical rulerships in astrology, and it was like I suddenly found the key to a code I had been trying to break. It was as if I was spontaneously coming out of a state of amnesia.

It had been sitting there in plain sight. So simple. So elegant.

Was this why my life fell apart? For this moment?

Astrology confirmed many things I knew about myself and helped me see qualities and possibilities that I had previously dismissed. I was born in the Aries season. Aries rules the head, so maybe that was another reason I loved the ventricles of the brain, deep inside of our heads. I am very heady. I love to learn. My credential collection was an expression of the strong Aries signature in my horoscope, with my Sun, Moon, Mercury, and Chiron, the wounded healer, all passing through the constellation when I was born. My credential collection was also an expression of never feeling good enough, of looking for validation in what I knew. Mars rules Aries, and I had undoubtedly suppressed and questioned my inner hero for most of my life.

My mind was racing faster than I could type. It all worked. I pulled up an image of the hyoid bone, which sits on top of the larynx. Thoughts and ideas continued to swirl in my head.

It looks exactly like the symbol for Taurus. Gemini rules the lungs and arms, twin structures in the body, and the myth is about grief - the emotion Chinese medicine says we store in our lungs. The aortic arch is the same shape as the symbol for Leo, and Leo rules the heart. A woman's reproductive system looks like a Scorpion and a man's like Scorpio's other archetype, a snake. The head of the femur looks like Jupiter, with the circulatory vessels to it like the red spot. Saturn rules the bones, and concentric, Saturnian rings make up the substructure of long bones. Our feet are like fish flippers, like the two fish representing Pisces.

The archetypal equivalency was present for every sign and every planet, and the vagus nerve compression points I routinely treated were all at the intersection of two signs.

A few months earlier, I took a sharp turn into exploring cosmology in the body after reading Graham Hancock's *Fingerprints of the Gods* and learning that mythology was a mode of communicating scientific information. For example, the ancient Egyptian myth of Isis and Osiris has numbers of the Earth's precessional cycle in it. They expressed cosmology through storytelling, not as we do today, through technical writing. I instantly had a thought only a physical or occupational therapist would be likely to have. *The earth is currently at approximately a twenty-three and one-half degree tilt. What anatomical structures are 23.5 degrees from the midline of the body?*

On a hunch, I pulled out my son's protractor for school. I measured the angle on the base of the skull between the jugular foramen, where the spinal cord exits the skull, and the jugular foramen, where the vagus nerve transitions from the cranial cavity. Twenty-three and one-half degrees crossed the jugular foramen! The earth's axial tilt varies from 22.1 to 24.5 degrees over many thousands of years, and those angles also crossed the opening. No matter what the axial tilt of the earth, the vagus nerve aligned with it.

I knew from physical therapy school that normal rotation between the first and second cervical vertebrae, C1, and C2, was forty-seven degrees to each side, twenty-three and one-half doubled! I always thought that was an odd number to be a standard value, as, in most of our books, average values were usually multiples of five. I knew other angles that matched the earth's axial tilt or were an even fraction or multiple of it. For example, the anterior cruciate ligament sits in the knee at an average forty-seven-degree angle of inclination. Given the number of dizziness, neck pain, and knee patients, the relevance of this alignment felt big. I knew other angles that related to the numbers in the myth of Isis and Osiris.

Decompressing the vagus nerve at the base of the skull is very much like putting someone back on their axis. The vagus nerve goes all the way from the brainstem to the pelvis, innervates the vocal cords, heart, and digestive system, gives sensory inputs from almost every organ to your brain, and uses the same neurotransmitter as muscles. For many years, I had logically used cranial decompression techniques for the vagus nerve to successfully treat patients with pain regardless of the location in the body as well as anxiety, depression, hallucinations, heart palpitations, and constipation. The vagus nerve is the most significant component of our parasympathetic nervous system, which helps us regulate our stress responses.

Stress and trauma always affect the voice and the breath. In the moments of stress and trauma, our breath changes, most often getting faster. We scream or sob or call for help. We lose our carefree arm swing and move our trunks like a block of wood. The vagus nerve can get stuck at the diaphragm, the muscle we breathe with, and the vocal cords, the muscles we speak with, and other places where anatomical structures go horizontally in the body, such as the base of the skull and the pelvic floor. Horizontal structure dysfunction in other areas of the body will also trigger a stress response and "lower the volume" of the vagus nerve. In my experience, knee and foot pain and biomechanics always responded very well to vagus nerve decompression at the base of the skull.

My oldest son used to delay going to sleep by coming out of his room to tell me that he had an elevated first rib, and I needed to correct it for him to go to sleep. An elevated first rib is a sign that the vagus nerve is compressed at the base of the skull. Treatment at the base of the skull almost always resolves a myriad of upper rib issues. This time, I delayed his bedtime, testing his first rib and other joints for restrictions and feeling for the astrological archetypes in the body while lying in bed. His first rib test on the right was positive. I knelt on the floor and put his head in my hands to check his cranial rhythmic impulse and feel for the ram's horns in his head, the symbol for the Aries constellation. They felt as if they were asymmetrical. The right side was distorted, feeling somewhat uncurled, and bent off toward the right. I held his Aries ram's horns in my mind's eye and my hands. I applied my myofascial technique, the one I developed myself. I found it much more efficient than other techniques I knew. It looked good in my mind's eye and felt symmetrical in my hands. I repeated the first rib test on each side. It was completely normal.

I let my oldest son go to sleep and repeated the process with my younger son. There was nothing to treat. Next, I repeated it with my husband, also an Aries. His ram's horns were distorted differently, with different positive biomechanical tests. Still, resolving the distortion in the ram's horns gave me the same biomechanical results that I got from the hands-on techniques I had used for years faster and more efficiently.

I continued to contemplate what was happening. The Aries warrior was not sitting right on top of the Taurus bull. Mars is the hero. Taurus represents desires. The tension is between the hero and the desires. It's also within the hero. If these were two other anatomical structures, I would say that they are sheared and creating compression or tension in the structures between them.

Would this technique work with everyone? How does a hero get sheared?

Using a form of energy medicine I now call Weller Schematics™, I spent several years validating how to restore alignment for the hero and all other archetypes within the body with clients in-person and online. Our alignment is not just within our body; it extends to the cosmos. A cosmology-based approach to the human body is like speaking to the body in its original language, creating rapid and lasting improvement in health, performance, and genius. It does not work at the expense of any other conventional and medically necessary approaches. On the contrary, it amplifies the positive effects. Below is an exercise to help you assess your inner warrior, your hero. You can find out more about my process and supporting research at https://melanieweller.com.

THE MEDICINE

The hero's journey is a universal story that lives through each of us. The head reveals clues as to the status of our inner hero. When the bridge to our inner hero needs repair, it can show up as mental health issues, physical pain, or both. You can find video instructions for this exercise and more at https://melanieweller.com/sacred-medicine.

Storytelling is one of the oldest healing tools. Mythology was a mode of bridging scientific information with everyday meaning to ensure it was remembered for generations. Likewise, we can use ancient storytelling paradigms in conjunction with our modern medicine, taking patients on the neurological superhighway to transformation. Here is part of my PYRAMIDS™ process.

Physical Tests: Here are three ways to measure head function and test your inner hero. All testing is to stay within pain-free limits. If you have any medical issues or concerns, check with your healthcare professionals before doing the tests.

1. Cervical Range of Motion Test: Find a horizontal line (real or imaginary) on the wall that is about eye level that you can use as a reference. See how far you can turn your head to each side, keeping your eyes following that line to keep you from compensatory movements. Typical rotation is 80 degrees to each side.

2. C1-C2 Test: Look down toward the floor, approximately 45-50 degrees. Find a similar horizontal reference line as you did above. Rotate your head slowly to each side. You should be able to go about 45 degrees to each side. If you feel like you "hit a brick wall" or go over a "speed bump" as you move, do not go further.

3. Rotation-Lateral Flexion Test: Turn the head as far as comfortable to one side. Leading with the ear that faces forward, bring that ear toward the chest. The normal range of motion is to be able to tilt the head forward approximately 45 degrees. A positive test involves minimal or asymmetrical movement.

Personal Inventory: Ask yourself the following questions.

1. Where are you acting as the hero in someone else's story at the expense of your own?

2. What is your superpower, and are you using it?

3. If you could remove one obstacle in your life, what would it be?

4. When you were a child, did you have to function much like an adult?

How did it feel to read and answer these questions? Simply asking these questions can improve the test results, especially if you had an emotional response.

Put your hero into thought, word, and action! How does your inner hero dress? Add some good detail. Do they wear a crown? Shoes? Jewelry? Now imagine you are wearing it! This approach works because metaphor activates the sensory cortex, which is where pain can exit. Next, determine the sound of your superpower. Maybe it is like the swoosh of the lightsaber or an electrical buzz. Perhaps Prince's *Purple Rain* plays when you arrive on the scene. Make that sound at least three times for as long as you can, up to 13 seconds. This approach works because the vagus nerve innervates the vocal cords. Singing and sounding are beneficial to reducing stress and inflammation - even singing in your head helps!

Imagine that you are dressed like your inner hero. Spend a moment getting yourself lined up with this image. Line up your eyes, heart, breath, and feet with your hero's. Now start moving *as* them. This approach works because the brain doesn't see doing something and imagining doing something differently. Plus, it's fun to move like your inner hero, even if it's just raising your eyebrows as they do!

Now retest yourself. What is better? How much better is it? What is still limited? You might have to repeat this practice and make a more extensive inquiry to get your desired results. Finally, post a photo of you with your hero's story and tag me on Facebook, Instagram, or Twitter @embodyyourstar!

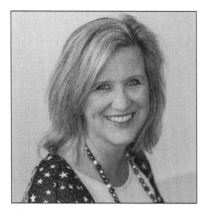

Melanie Weller is a Medical Visionary and author whose upcoming book, *The Bridge Between Your Story and Your Body*, describes her paradigm-shifting process for healthcare professionals to amplify healing, increase compliance, and accelerate outcomes in their patients by bridging storytelling and medicine. Melanie uses the vagus nerve as a portal to bring over 25 years of experience to her leading-edge systems, grounding cosmology, story, and intuition in the body. Melanie teaches healthcare professionals and performance experts how to enhance their existing practices to help their patients measurably overcome physical limitations and transcend mental health issues. Melanie is a Physical Therapist, Board-Certified Orthopedic Clinical Specialist, Certified Athletic Trainer, and Certified Exercise Expert for Aging Adults. She also co-authored a sleep course for continuing education credits for the American Physical Therapy Association. Melanie lives on the parade route in New Orleans, Louisiana with her husband, her two children, and her German Shepherd. She is almost an empty nester!

CHAPTER 3

AWAKEN YOUR INNER DRAGON

HOW TO CONNECT TO YOUR SOURCE OF POWER

Atlantis Wolf

"Powerlessness and silence go together."

-Margaret Atwood

Only one of my dragon spirit guides was birthed through my physical body, the first one, the red one. He gestated as I endured 41 years of rage, savagery, and verbal cruelty that I answered with silence. Like an oak tree whose new shoots are cut down to the ground when it reaches for the sun in spring, I grew deeper and deeper roots into my silent interior, reaching for spiritual sustenance and cultivating gardens and landscapes to roam and live safe and alone. I didn't know spiritual beings lived there, too, until the dragon arrived in a spectacular, blazing burst of authority, showing me how to speak with power, not brutishness or malice.

MY STORY

"You sound like a bitch," my dad said.

He was in the driver's seat of our family's gray Dodge Caravan, dusty with dirt from the single-lane country road where we lived as he and I drove into town to the bicycle shop to get a new chain.

The windows were down, so he yelled his reply back to me. But he had a loud voice, no need to yell.

He asked what I would do when we got back. I answered that I was going to ride my bicycle to my best friend's house and listen to records. I was wearing my favorite rainbow-striped t-shirt and red shorts, hot and dusty, sitting in the shadow of the back seat with my broken bicycle on the sunny summer day. I said nothing. I was 11 years old, my dad 31.

"I think it's the new friends you have at school," he said. "They probably sound bitchy, too."

That was my dad's favorite game, ask you a simple, superficial question and pierce your answer until he found the liquid core. Next, wound you, then step on the wound until you felt the ooze.

My parents married young and graduated from college with two kids. They moved to the country to live a simple life at a time in America when that was a popular notion. My mom grew up in the inner city of an industrial city, my dad in a comfortable metropolitan suburb of a smaller but similar working-class city. I wanted to grow up on Sesame Street.

In school, I loved reading, writing, and recess. My eyes would move from the chalkboard to the window at every opportunity. In sixth grade, I won second place for a poem about drifting from the solar system out into space. In my senior year of high school, I told my dad I wanted to major in English.

He pulled out the Sunday newspaper, classified section.

"Do you see any advertisements for an English major?" he said. "No, because there are none. Look for engineering jobs. Lots to choose. That's where the jobs are." I said nothing, holding the red damask couch pillow in my lap.

I'll take English electives every semester in addition to my engineering classes. He won't know.

Full-time college students are required to take 12 credits per semester. Engineering students need 18 per semester to graduate in four years. I started with 21. I graduated with enough credits for a dual degree in Civil Engineering and English with a minor in Environmental Engineering.

My parents and my brother came to my college commencement. The sun was shining as we walked from lunch to the auditorium. I was in heels, a white dress, red lipstick, and a black cap and gown.

"You know," my dad said as we walked to the ceremony, "I always thought you'd lose weight when you got to college."

I said nothing.

I'm glad I took that job three states away. I'm going to miss my mom.

I moved to Baltimore and met my future husband, who lost his job when his company was bought out by a conglomerate. We moved to Chicago for four years, then back to my hometown to get married and begin a family. Two kids later, my mom became terminally ill, and my husband left, moving to the other side of the city.

It was the year after my mom died. I made plans to take my kids for their first visit to my family's house in the Caribbean. The financial hurdle was always plane tickets. My dad purchased our tickets and said he and his girlfriend would be at the house only for the first day, for "an elegant transition," It was to be the first time I had a vacation in five years.

"I'm calling to talk about the trip," he said two weeks before we were leaving. "When are you coming?"

You bought the tickets. You know when we're coming. Ask your travel agent. She sent them six months ago.

I was sitting in my red house in my downstairs office off the living room, the one I rebuilt from a side porch with three walls of window screens to a solid room with windows front and back for privacy. My kids were in bed. I was checking emails and taking his call with the door closed. My sleep deficit was about three hours per night.

I had worked all day as a business analyst for a bank job by the airport 45 minutes from home. I had worked for eight months watching the airplanes take off from the runway. My office window was facing the end, so I never saw them landing, only launching. Every day. For hours. *One day, I'll take a plane and go to a peaceful place.*

"Me and the kids are coming in on the fifth and leaving on the ninth," I said.

"Well, you know we've already been here for two months, so we're good," he said. "We haven't bought our tickets back yet, but we're thinking if we leave on the eighth, that will give us time to spend with your kids, and then you can have some time together as a family, too."

I said nothing. My skin began to get prickly, the way skin does when it's burned by the midday sun, unprotected. My heart began to thump in a lumpy way, the way it did since I was a child and unable to answer my dad's attacks in a masterful or meaningful way. The organs in my abdomen felt crushed as if a giant's hand had squeezed them in his fist.

"But you said you guys were leaving the day we got there," I said. "What changed?"

"This is my house!" he said. "I don't have to accommodate you!"

My prickly skin became hotter as if curls of flame were traveling along the surface from my feet and hands up to my throat. The bowl of bone between my hips felt like a cauldron. The sound of burning logs, sparking and crackling in the night air, filled my ears. The tears forming in my eyes turned hard and red. With the phone to my ear, I inhaled and lifted my lips to the sky as a fully gestated dragon with red scales and emerald green eyes was birthed from my cauldron up and out of my mouth. It felt like a portal opened near my tailbone, and a ball of flaming lava pushed through my body in one ring-of-fire push.

"I AM ALLOWED TO ASK QUESTIONS!" I said. "I AM ALLOWED TO KNOW WHAT IS HAPPENING TO ME! I AM ALLOWED TO DECIDE WHAT I DO WITH MY KIDS!"

I am allowed to speak my opinion.

I am allowed to make my plans.

I am allowed to be alone with my kids.

I am allowed to rest and cry and grieve for my mother.

I am allowed to be.

I am allowed.

I am allowed.

I allow myself to be.

The dragon's skin was steaming from the birth by fire as he curled around me so close that I felt his scales on all sides and his heat. Surrounded by his massive, masculine musculature, I felt protected, safe, and warm. My breathing was heavy, steady. I felt logical and large. My entire body was vibrating with electricity. *Did he speak, or did I?*

"You can't tell me when to leave my house," my dad said.

I hung up the phone.

I left my job as a business analyst to earn a license as a massage therapist a year after my mom died. No one would hire me out of school, so I became an entrepreneur. I would save money and find affordable retreats to explore my vast interior landscape. I saw the Archangel Gabriel in the events around my mom's death. After her death, I often saw spirit guides around my clients, usually at the end of sessions. My practice focused on pain because there was often psychic pain intertwined with the experience of physical pain. When I used my hands, the spirits would guide them to places that helped ease my client's pain. I wanted to ease my pain as well.

At a weekend women's retreat, I was lying on a mat and led into a guided meditation. I saw my dad and me on a green grassy knoll on a sunny day facing each other. We were locked in battle. My left hand was covered in a metal mitt. Imagine your hand holding the clapper of a bell, and the bell is surrounding your hand and wrist but locked in place so you can't release your fingers; your whole hand is encased inside. At the top of the mitt was a heavy chain connected to the same shape on my dad's hand. My left hand was chained to his right.

He had a metal helmet over his head, something you would see on a knight, but the eye screen was black, covered inside by a black material, blocking his ability to see. He was angry, cursing and yelling, pulling his hand in quick bursts so that I almost fell to my knees with each violent yank. I arrived in this angry deadlock not speaking. After pausing to understand what I was seeing, I looked at my left hand and dissolved the lock with my mind, attaching the metal mitt to his left hand. He continued to struggle at the locks and chain, lurching and pitching his body down the other side of the hill. I watched him fight himself until he was gone, and I was standing in the sun feeling the breeze on the grass across my bare legs, still and silent.

As I continued my medical massage practice and path of self-discovery, I began to see animal guides around my clients and more dragons in a circle around me as I stood or sat in meditation on my medicine wheel. I knew I would face my dad again.

At a retreat in Sedona, I was lying on a mat in a guided meditation and saw my dad and I facing each other again, this time on a wide-open plain. I had enormous white angel wings outstretched, with a short white dress, gold sandals, and a long sword with a gold hilt. I was hovering ten feet off the ground with everyone my dad had wounded behind me: my mother, my brother, my maternal grandmother, my kids, and a group of approximately 50 people I didn't immediately know by name.

My dad was alone with a large black demon on his back, covering my dad's eyes with his left hand and covering my dad's right hand, which held the hilt of a silver sword. The demon initiated each thrust of the sword; my dad couldn't see me. I was actively fighting my dad, whose body was shielding the demon from harm while protecting the people with my wings. As we battled each other, it became obvious I had only one option. I plunged the sword through my dad's body, pushing the demon off him, holding his wriggling body at the tip of my sword.

"Dad!" I said. "Turn around! I can't keep him there forever."

My dad was poised between the demon and me. He saw me, saw the crowd behind my wings, and turned to see the demon behind him.

"You have to kill him," I said. "I can't. He belongs to you."

He looked at the sword in his hand and looked up at me.

"But without him," he said, "I have no power."

The ting-shahs chimed; the guided meditation ended. I sat and cried for my dad, wondering when he would meet his demon and win. I walked outside to see the sunset on the red rocks of Sedona with a council of dragons around me.

The red dragon never left his post as my guardian. Occasionally, if my dad was up to his tricks, the dragon would smile, open one eye and let the smoke drift out of his nostrils as if to say, *Do I need to wake up?* I haven't needed to wake him up yet, but I love feeling him around me.

THE MEDICINE

If you are reading this, you have a sleeping dragon inside you. You are being called to awaken that dragon, face what you fear that lives in your shadow, and stand in your power. When you stand in your circle of power, you are not aggressive or cruel; you create a space for your whole being to exist in the world. Dragons are an archetype for personal power. They represent cosmic balance and being fully realized as a being composed of equal light and shadow.

If you would like me to walk through this meditation with you, go to my YouTube channel: https://youtu.be/u6mkhCzIZ_E

Prepare a solitary space that is comfortable outside and find a powerful being, a tree that is so big you can't put your arms around it, the ocean, a river wider than your body, a rock big enough for three people to sit on it. Sit with your back against the tree, stand and gaze at the ocean or river. Sit comfortably on the rock. Silence your phone.

Take three breaths in through your nose and out of your mouth as if emptying your body of all thoughts, expectations, and future appointments. With each exhale, relax into the tree, or soften your gaze into the water or sink into the rock. Exhale slower and longer each time, settling your body and allowing the air, land, and water to embrace you.

Call to the four directions: your birth (East), your present moment (South), your future death (West), and your ancestors and spirit guides (North). Ask your higher power to hold a space of love and protection for you, surrounding you with golden light.

You are about to meet your dragon for the first time. Greet them with wonder and curiosity. Imagine all the details of the dragon surrounding you, wrapping itself around you.

How big is it?

What color is its skin?

What color are its eyes?

Does it have scales or feathers?

Is it a land dragon or a water dragon? Ask your dragon if you don't know.

Imagine you are reaching out to touch it. How does it feel? Is it warm or cool?

Extend your senses and imagine yourself feeling what it's like to be the dragon.

Breathe with your dragon.

Take time to merge.

When you feel ready, imagine the person who holds power against you. Who are you not allowed to criticize? Who does not allow you to speak your opinion? Who keeps you silent? That person is in front of you. Imagine what they are wearing, how they are standing or sitting. Bring every detail to life until they are a clear vision in your mind.

With your dragon around you and your clear vision of a person, begin humming. Breathe in through your nose and hum with your exhale, not a high-pitch hum through the top of your nose, a low-tone hum that comes from your belly, your golden bowl, your cauldron, and feels like your whole abdomen is humming. If your hum begins at the tip of your nose, imagine it traveling down to your lower abdomen with each exhale. Continue until you feel the hum vibrating from your throat down to your belly.

You embody power. Speak out loud to the person who holds power against you. Tell them how you feel. Allow all emotions and opinions to move out of your body and into the air, sending them to the vision of the person in front of you. You control the conversation.

Imagine the other person speaking back to you. Reach out to the dragon. Continue speaking with your words, your voice, and your power. Feel the tree, the water, or the rock supporting you. Feel the protection of golden light holding you. Speak until you have no words. Scream, spit or cry if the emotions can't find the words of expression. Keep going until you feel empty.

When it's time, come back to the present. Give yourself time to reflect and bring back the experience. Write about what you heard, saw, and felt in a journal. Drink water. Allow the experience to sit in your body. Stay quiet and listen for more messages from other spiritual guides around you.

You are the sacred medicine speaking into the world. Everything you need to heal and ascend into your next spiritual evolution exists within you. Awaken your dragon. Embrace your shadow. Stand in your power.

I'm Atlantis Wolf. And I believe in you.

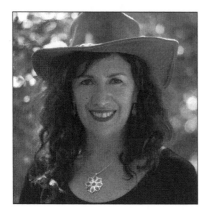

Atlantis Wolf is a Shamanic Life Coach and workshop leader who helps people seeking answers to their medical, spiritual, and emotional questions with the help of her spirit guides, power animals, and galactic dragons.

She grew up on a single-lane dirt road in the country, walking barefoot through the forest, whistling to birds, and wondering what she was supposed to do on Earth. As a child, she sat under the back porch awning and tape-recorded a thunderstorm so she could listen to it as she fell asleep. At an early age, she realized sound is medicine.

She lives like an oak tree with an equal number of branches reaching up to the light as those reaching down into the darkness - an equal amount of living above ground holding coaching sessions, workshops, and shamanic breathwork events, as below ground cultivating a vast interior landscape of gardens and spiritual healing temples. Her stories are in direct proportion to above as below. There are stories below her stories.

She has worked as a civil engineer, technical writer, business analyst, project manager, licensed medical massage therapist, marketing consultant, and entrepreneur. Below the ground, she was spiritually asleep until her mother's death awakened her gifts to see and communicate with spiritual beings and remember her past lives as an Egyptian healer, Toltec curandera, and Ayurvedic traveling shaman. She is the Dragon Medicine Woman.

Atlantis is a single mom with four kids and five cats. She lives on Turtle Island.

AtlantisWolf.com

DragonMedicineWoman@gmail.com

YouTube: Atlantis Wolf

CHAPTER 4

MANIFESTATION 101: ALIGNMENT

TAKING INSPIRED ACTIONS TO CREATE DESIRED OUTCOMES

Aliesha B. Davis, M.Ed.

If simply wanting something—writing it down and putting a picture of it on a board—is all one had to do to manifest, I would not have written this chapter, and you probably would not be reading it. However, the ideal premise behind vision boards and the surface level of understanding the Law of Attraction will have you believe otherwise.

MY STORY

In the Beginning…

From the time I can remember, I always felt I was special, destined for something, but I was not sure what. As a child, I was always drawn to the sky, sun, and artsy-type things. Then as I got older and influences around me, from parents to peers to society in general, I began to let go of or get away from what I loved, enjoyed, and centered me, which was creating and being a dreamer. I allowed myself to be put into a box and tried very hard to do everything that went along with the label on the box. From about eleven to twenty-nine, I was boxed in by parameters, standards, and expectations I allowed to be placed on me that I thought I wanted until I realized I didn't. Now what?

Lights, Camera, Action...

I was a "good girl," whatever that's supposed to mean, but that is the box label and image I was portraying. I was brought up in a middle-class neighborhood, had all of my needs taken care of, and most of my wants. My parents were respected in the community and leaders in our church. I was an average student and living a pretty average teenage life. I got a used car at sixteen that was upgraded to a new car for graduation. Then off to college I went. With great excitement, I was out of my parent's house and semi on my own. At eighteen, I knew it all and was off to conquer the world.

My boyfriend was coming to the same college, and it was all good to me. Things at college were going great, classes were good, social life good, I'm good. I decided I would not spend the night with my boyfriend because that did not look right according to my box label. Now that's not to say we were not having sex because we were getting it on on a regular basis and had been for around four years. However, that was behind closed doors, and the image remained intact. That worked out for about a month or less before I started staying at his apartment more than my dorm. It was official; I was grown in my mind. I was making grown-up moves and doing grown-up things, or so I thought. We were so in love and ready to conquer the world together. Since I was now living in another city, no one knew me, and my image was still intact, until I got pregnant.

Down the Rabbit Hole...

I was terrified to tell my mom I was pregnant. Oh yeah, I got pregnant at fifteen and had an abortion, so I was devastated to be back in this situation or to have to tell her because, once again, the image was intact. I told her, and her response was, "You are going to have to have this one." She told me I would have to tell my dad, and she told me I needed to get married. So at eighteen, when your mom tells you something, that means it is good advice, right? She would not tell me anything wrong, right? After all, parents have all the answers, right? Well, I've since learned there is so much gray area here. Anyway, as my mother advised, I got married to my junior high/middle school sweetheart, also a college student, and already had two children.

As you can see, I was going down the rabbit hole rapidly, but naïve and cluelessly forged full steam ahead. After all, the image was still intact because we were married and a young little family. I went from high school graduation in September of 1997 to wife and mom by September of 1998.

Deeper Down the Hole…

I had only seen one person be a wife and mom, and that was the example I patterned myself after. Never mind that she had a forty-one-year jump start over me. I now had a new box. So I stepped out of the good girl box into the wife and mom box with a new set of rules and labels. I wanted so badly to be the perfect wife and mom and to do all the things I thought and believed a perfect wife and mom should do and be. I had just turned nineteen and was very optimistic. I still believed I knew everything, and so I began my roles of wife and mom.

Life Happened…

I cannot really detail the next five to ten years of my life because they were a whirlwind. I had many experiences that accompanied the box I was presently in. I truly had the ups and downs, highs and lows, and joys and sorrows of what I had undertaken. Some of the most challenging, aside from the emotional aspects, was working full-time, going to school full-time, and for a brief moment working an additional part-time job as well. The constant migraine headaches should have been a warning that something was wrong, and I needed to reevaluate and reassess some things, but I told myself *mind over matter* and continued toward what I thought a successful life looked like. I got my degree and started my teaching career. I would finally be happy, right? This is what I should be doing, right? Oh, this is the perfect time to grow our family, right? So I stopped taking my birth control to countless conversations with a hesitant and apprehensive husband on the idea of growing the family.

I got pregnant within two months of coming off of birth control, and by age twenty-five, I had my husband, two beautiful daughters, and a promising career. While I was steadily checking things off the box label sheet and things in my life on the surface appeared great; they were falling apart on the inside. I was so invested in the image and appearance that I just hoped and believed it would work itself out in reality. I could not come to grips with why I was not happy, why I was not fulfilled, and what I was doing wrong.

My husband seemed more unhappy than me, and we argued constantly. He wanted one thing, I wanted something totally different, and compromises were very limited. Still, from the outside, we appeared to be thriving. We bought a house and cars and dressed the part all under stress and financial strain. We were living paycheck to paycheck with enormous debt. From having to pawn jewelry and car titles to having utilities turned off for days or weeks at a time, we went through it all. Except for my mom, no one had a clue as to what was happening within this well-maintained bubble, and the image was still intact.

The arguments were almost daily and aggressive. I was verbally and emotionally abused and did not know or realize its effects on my children or me. I went to church, prayed, and wrote down things I wanted to see happen and come forth in my life, but it felt like the harder I tried, the worse things got. I was on such a roller coaster, very confused and depressed. I loved my husband, and at times we would click. I continued holding on to the hope that it would all get better. My hope kept me going and striving and pushing until, at some point, I realized nothing around me lined up with the things I was hoping for, and I became hopeless. This was probably the lowest point in my life. I will say with certainty hopelessness is the worst feeling I have experienced in my life. I felt like I was under a rock, and nothing I could come up with was going to get me from under it. My marriage became toxic and spilled over into other aspects of my life that made simple tasks very hard because I was miserable. However, I couldn't let anyone know or see that. So I worked even harder on making sure I looked a certain way, said the right things, my kids were well groomed and well-spoken, and everything looked picture perfect.

The Shift…

Little by little, I started being introduced to meditation and mindfulness through the OWN network and Super Soul Sunday. I started listening to spiritual leaders, Dr. Wayne Dyer and Dr. Deepak Chopra, and read their books. For the first time in my life, someone was giving me actions to do to get the things I wanted. I began to make shifts in my mindset and started to find my true and authentic self. At some point, I realized that I had learned to be a wife and mom. However, I had never learned to do me. In the midst and cycle of it all, I lost me, myself, and I. Now, slowly but surely, I began to learn about myself. I began being honest with myself, revealing some ugly truths in and about my life. I had to learn that I could trust myself and my decision-making. I had to learn to forgive myself for all the things I didn't know before I learned them. I had to learn to love me. I had to learn, believe, and affirm I am enough. I had to learn how to show up in the world as my true authentic self. Once I was able to stand in my truth, I freed myself from the burden of my box and the labels that came with it. I totally burst the box wide open and got the will to walk away from a marriage and life that was toxic and detrimental to me. I gained a new lease on life and learned to trust the process and enjoy the journey.

Revelations...

There is a saying I love, which states, "When the student is ready, the teacher will appear." So while getting answers to my questions, I have learned how to allow myself to receive and listen to a voice inside of me that is very subtle and almost like a whisper. Some may call it your gut. The problem is we're taught early and often not to listen to it, to vanquish it, or even try to reason and rationalize against the logic from it. Sometimes we do it to the point of it becoming suppressed or dormant. However, as I have continued to ask questions and ponder information, answers and solutions are revealed to me through life lessons, or a conversation I may overhear, a television program I'm watching, a song on the radio, or even a book I may read. I discovered the "me" I needed was present all along. I had to realize I was not a victim to my life, my circumstances, or the box I allowed myself to be placed in. I learned I was the designer and orchestrator of my life. I have and always had the power to call into being and form whatever I deemed myself worthy of and wanted. My situation had only been the catalyst to show me I was in control of my destiny. It showed me I had the power and right, but more importantly, the obligation to create my life, my story, and my journey as I see fit.

THE MEDICINE

The Law of Attraction is about manifestation, but there are 11 more Universal Laws, one of which is The Law of Inspired Action. It is the law of inspired action that aligns you with your desires and allows you to manifest desired outcomes over and over and over again. It's no secret; there is a formula:

(Mindset + Intentions = Magick), your thoughts plus inspired actions equate to you manifesting your heart's desire.

Inspired action comes from an internal nudge to do something, simply meaning you have an internal desire to do something. Inspired action is not a plan of action. It is not something you think about ahead of time where you create a list of steps to take. It is about you being intentional in listening and allowing the Universe to guide you, to give you that internal direction, and you following through on that guidance.

Here are some activities to do to help create the space and opportunities to go beyond the surface level of manifesting into alignment.

1. Get Clear on Where You Are

Ask yourself:

- Who am I?
- What do I believe about myself, and am I okay with it?
- What are the things I want to change?

2. What Do You Want?

Make a list of what you want. What are the desired outcomes you would like to manifest and call forth into your life?

3. Affirm, Affirm, Affirm

Tell yourself positive words, encouraging words, inspiring words, and motivating words to assure your mind, both conscious and subconscious are in agreement, and sending the correct message and frequency into the Universe.

Examples:

I am worthy

I am unlimited

I am powerful

I am enough

4. Focus on Solutions

Now that you are clear on where you are, where you want to go, and have created a path and frequency to align yourself with your desires, begin to become solution-based. For example, rather than saying, "I'm so tired today," focus on, "I feel really good and energized when I _____," or "when I'm able to _____." Or, "I'm going to _____, so I have more energy and feel good about myself and my situation." Basically, it's a mindset hack. So whatever situation has you in a negative or problematic space, approach it from the solution standpoint.

5. Take Inspired Action…Be Intentional

Whatever you want, focus your thoughts on what you believe will get you there. Think about actions you believe you need to do or the direction you want to go. Reflect back to where you are and where you want to go.

6. Live From a Place of Wholeness

You have identified where you are and what you want, making sure your head is in the game, opening the path to receive, and made moves toward the thing you want. Now you must visualize yourself with it. Engage all or as many of the senses as possible. What does it taste like, look like, smell like, feel like, sound like? Close your eyes, go deep within, and truly allow yourself to be in the moment. In this moment, there are only possibilities, an infinite field of possibilities that are yours to have, to hold, and to savor.

7. Gratefulness

In number six, you lived from the place of possibilities and experienced the very thing you desire. Now, be grateful for it. Be grateful from the space and place where you felt the magick. Be grateful from the place of pure potential and possibilities. Be grateful at your core for not just what is coming but also for all that is already yours.

This is not a one-and-done activity or process. This is just a start and guidance in helping you open up to yourself. If you would like to continue this work, join my Let's J.A.M. 21 Day Challenge in journaling, affirming, and meditating your way into shifting your mindset and getting into alignment in order to define and design your destiny at www.CreatingHappy.me

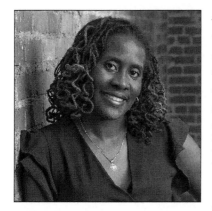

Aliesha Bibbins Davis is a lightworker, creative spirit, and truth seeker. She is the mother of three daughters and a twenty-one-year veteran educator. She is a certified life coach specializing in mindset and manifestation and a Reiki practitioner. Aliesha teaches individuals how to go from where they are to where they want to be.

Aliesha is also the founder and owner of Creating Happy, L.L.C., which is the platform she uses to teach others how to trust the process and enjoy the journey of pursuing their passion, living with purpose, and defining and designing their destiny.

CHAPTER 5

AMPLIFY YOUR INNER WISDOM

MANIFEST YOUR SOULMATE

Sarah Sparks

"Whatever you desire, no matter what it is, will eventually come to you."

-Sarah Sparks

MY STORY

By the time you finish this chapter, I want you to feel at home, whatever that means to you. I want you to know you are special, unique, loved, and blessed. You are meant for more. There's no more hurting or pain. There's trust, freedom, safety, benevolence, love, acceptance, and peace awaiting you. Just keep going. You are created for this. Don't give up. I believe in you. Just know, you are meant for more.

I haven't always listened to my inner wisdom. I was 18 years old. I felt overwhelmed, tired, pulled in many different directions. I was having a hard time making decisions. I felt like the weight of the world was on my shoulders. I felt like I had to make all of life's major decisions in a short amount of time, and I felt like time was running out to make those decisions.

I was raised Catholic and was not taught to have a relationship with Divine, Spirit, or God. I was taught to pray for others who were sick, dying, or at war; something had to be wrong to chat with God. Nothing was wrong in my life, so why would I pray and ask for help?

One night I had enough of my swirling thoughts and not knowing the answers to life's major decisions. So, I prayed to God. Before I went to sleep, I said, "God, show me what I am to do with my life. Show me in a dream. However, you want to show me. Just show me. Please. I need your help."

That night I had what I call "The Dream". I was walking along the beach. White sand and sharp seashells crunched beneath my feet. The seagulls were flying overhead. I felt the wet, salty air on my face. The sun was setting. The vast, clear, open water was to my right. The sun was to my right. I was walking along the beach. Everything felt so right. Perfect. I looked up, and ahead of me was a man. He had a tan neck, dark brown hair, and broad shoulders. He was six feet tall. I remember thinking in the dream; *oh look, that man is taller than me! Yes! God, you did good!* Everything in this dream: the man, beach, sunset, salty air—everything felt like home. It felt like this was right where I was to be. This was my home. He was my home. I was my home. In this place, I am home. And then, I woke up.

I had The Dream once a week for an entire year. I awoke each time, knowing this was the answer to my prayer. This place, this man, and how I was feeling were the answer to my prayer.

Yet I thought, *could it be that simple? I allowed God in. I asked for what I wanted. And I received an answer. Was it really that simple?*

The problem was I didn't trust myself. I didn't trust the answer. I thought life had to be much harder, more complicated than simply allowing, asking, and receiving. Because I believed it had to be much harder, The Universe, God, Spirit responded with, "Your wish is my command. You want a harder life, so it is." And it was until I learned to follow my inner wisdom.

What shifted for me to begin listening to my inner wisdom? Well, nine years went by from the time I had The Dream until I truly began listening to my inner wisdom. During that time, I married a man I knew I wasn't in love with, and I knew I was not to marry. He was not the man from The Dream. I went to a graduate school I was told (by my inner wisdom) not to go to. I took jobs I knew were not the right fit for me.

What I discovered after I reviewed my decisions and life is every time I said "No" and didn't trust my inner wisdom, the further away I got from the true me, the real me. I felt my soul lose a piece of itself. The more I didn't listen to my inner wisdom, the further down the hole I went into depression, despair, and disappointment in myself.

I got to a point where I planned my death. It was at that time that something shifted in me. I was two weeks away from ending my life when I met a young 16-year-old girl named Hannah. In one week, I "ran into her" at a hair salon, the tanning salon, and she was my waitress at a local pizza parlor. I picked up the local newspaper a few days after our various "run-ins" and saw a write-up of her in the newspaper. The article listed all of her accomplishments, and I was in awe. It felt like I was looking at and reading about a younger version of myself. That is when I realized I was in the obituary section of the newspaper. Hannah had taken her life between the Sunday she was my waitress and when the newspaper was printed, which was four days.

Right there, as I held the newspaper, I heard God say, "Sarah, you're meant for more."

At that moment, everything shifted for me. I knew if someone else, God/Source/Creator, saw something in me and knew I was meant for more, I could find a way to believe in me too.

Incrementally, not all at once, I began shifting everything about my life. I knew there was something inside me wanting to be extraordinary, have a voice, and to be shared with the world. I didn't know what it was. I didn't know anything about my soul's calling, my inner wisdom, nor my gifts. All I knew was I was meant for more.

A friend recognized that the shifts and changes I was making in my life weren't easy. So, as a great friend does, she asked me to go on vacation with her to St. Pete Beach, Florida. After being told three different times to go to Mulligan's, a restaurant and bar, we went. While there, I had to go to the bathroom. On my way, I walked past a bearded man in tan cargo shorts, a blue-gray t-shirt, flip flops, a baseball cap, and glasses. Something inside of me hopped. It felt like part of me knew him. I ignored the feeling and continued to the bathroom.

I walked back to my table, and the bearded man strolled over to me and said, "You don't smile much, do ya?"

His odd pickup line intrigued me and pissed me off. After a few minutes of small talk, the bearded man said, "May I offer you and your friend a rape-free drive back to your hotel?"

Friend, he had me there. I felt safe, plus he'd save me the cab fare back to our hotel; great logic, right?!

I didn't want him to know where we were staying, so we got a drink and walked along the beach to chat it up a bit more. As we were walking, I dropped my cup. "Shoot, I don't want the birds to get it," I said, and he continued walking.

I turned around and there it was: The Dream. I was walking along the beach. White sand and sharp seashells crunched beneath my feet. The seagulls were flying overhead. I felt the wet, salty air on my face. The sun was setting. The vast, clear, open water was to my right. The sun was to my right. I was walking along the beach. Everything felt so right. Perfect. I looked up, and ahead of me was a man. He had a tan neck, dark brown hair, and broad shoulders. He was six feet tall.

Friend, meet Mr. Craig Sparks, my husband, father of our two daughters, and my soulmate. Right then and there, I knew I was home. I began listening to my inner wisdom and continue to amplify it every day. Now, I share with you the medicine that changed my life around for good.

THE MEDICINE

What do you do if you want to have the experiences I had (and continue to have)? What could you do to have the experience of manifesting your soulmate? How could you get the sexy lover of your dreams? How do you get the clarity and the knowing of, "Yes, this is going to work out for me?"

So many people have done this process, used it, worked it, and allowed it to work for them. So much so that they met their soulmate, and then I got to officiate their marriage. It was just so much fun!

What I did (and I didn't know I was doing it): November of 2003, I had this feeling I really needed to know what I wanted in a husband. I got married to my ex-husband in August 2004. So, in November of 2003, months before I was to be married to my now ex-husband, I wrote out everything I wanted in a husband. After I was done, I thought, *I don't think this man I am going to marry is the man for me and I need to tell him that. It is better now than later.*

The ex-husband and I met up at my parents' place. We didn't have a place together yet because I was still in college. We sat in my parents' kitchen, on the floor, underneath the stovetop burners in November of 2003. I turned to him and said, "Alright, I got to tell you something, and I have to show you this. I wrote out this list of everything I want in a husband. I don't think it is you. I don't want you to change. I don't want you to try to become this person. Because I don't think that naturally, you are this person."

He responded, "Oh no. I can. I can be this person."

I expressed, "I am sure, but then you aren't honoring who you are. I… I… I don't think you are this person. It's not that there is anything wrong with you. I just had this aha moment, and I don't think I should marry you. And you are not the husband I want to marry. I think we should just be done."

"Oh no, no, no, no. We can work it out," he pleaded.

I ended up marrying him in August of 2004. Fast forward to 2009; I was starting to move out and packing everything up. I found the wedding planner in the bottom of the dresser drawer. In the planner, I found the list I wrote back in November of 2003 outlining what I wanted in a husband. All the reasons why I was leaving were on this list because he was not that man.

And then, I met the man from that list, the same man from The Dream, who you now know is Mr. Craig Sparks, my husband, my soulmate, and father of our two daughters!

Therefore, the first step to take is to really know what you want in a partner. Write out everything you want in your partner (husband/wife/life partner). To do this, ask yourself the following questions:

- How do I want to be treated?
- What are the experiences I want to have?
- How do I want to feel in this relationship?
- How do I want to feel being my true self in this relationship?
- What are the conversations I am having?
- Where are we going together?
- What does our morning look like?
- What does our afternoon and evening look like?
- Do we work together or not?
- Do we travel together?
- What does my soulmate, sexy lover look like?
- How am I appreciated in this relationship?
- How am I loved?
- How am I respected?
- What else am I missing that I want in my soulmate?

Clear your mind and let go of any expectations you think others have over you. Let go of any assumptions you have in your mind. Go into your heart. Write a letter to God/Spirit/The Universe about everything you want in your ideal sexy soulmate relationship. Do not hold anything back. Make your requests as specific as you want. The clearer you are in your request, the clearer God/Spirit/The Universe is on what you want. This way, God/Spirit/The Universe can then go to work on your behalf to bring what you desire to you.

Now, here's what you have to do next. You must allow God/Spirit/The Universe to go to work on your behalf. To symbolize you letting go of the control on how your soulmate is going to come into your life, you will burn the letter. See the ashes blow away in the wind, allowing your requests to be delivered to The Universe.

The final step is for you to act as if you are already in this relationship now. BE the person you want to be in this relationship now. Why is this important? When you are being the vibration of what you desire, that desire has no other option but to come to you.

Here's what I know: whatever you desire, no matter what it is, will eventually come to you. When it does, it will happen all of a sudden and feel out of the blue. It will feel easy, effortless, and enjoyable. Yet you've been planning, creating, and have become who you have needed to be to allow this desire to come to you! It all starts with you knowing you are meant for more, asking for what you really want, allowing it to come to you, and you becoming who you have needed to be.

Write your letter today! You are special, unique, loved, and blessed. I believe in you. You are created for this. Don't give up. Just know, you are meant for more. I love and honor you. Cheers to you manifesting your soulmate!

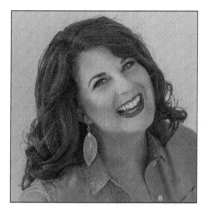

Sarah Sparks is the Spiritual Director at *Create the Spark, LLC.* Sarah is a farm-raised, college-educated, former local government employee turned business owner who is no longer ashamed of her spiritual woo-woo-ness. She guides fun, fabulous, fashionable females to lead with their souls by listening to their inner wisdom. Sarah believes you have limitless power to lead with your soul and listen to your inner wisdom, and she can help you tap into that. Let's do this! Visit https://www.sarahsparks.love to receive Sarah's FREE guide, *Amplify Your Inner Wisdom: Manifest Your Dream Partner and Life*

CHAPTER 6

THE MAKING OF AN EMPATH

HOW TRAUMA MOLDS THE SENSITIVE SOUL

Morrighan Lynne

MY STORY

My family was a ragtag group of dysfunctional souls. I suppose it would be the mature thing to say that my parents tried their best, but sometimes I'm not so sure. My mother was a covert narcissist who had a propensity for using manipulation and guilt/shame tactics to get her way. My stepfather expressed himself through angry outbursts and infantile tantrums when he didn't feel respected as the man of the house. I learned to stay out of their way, keep to myself, and become the young people-pleaser that inevitably develops in these environments.

Neither of my parents seemed to be able to handle their money wisely, causing us to move more times than I can count. I attended thirteen schools in my first seven years, crafting me to be a master of chameleonism. I could shape and shift like a pro. I was the water, molding to the container I was poured into, whether I liked it or not. As a child, I didn't know it was wrong. It was my life. I just went along with it, doing my best to make friends and reinventing myself from school to school.

When I was ten, my little body started to change, and my stepfather started to notice. In a flash of a moment, I went from a bright-eyed innocent child to being acutely aware of prying eyes with dirty intentions. I woke up to the dangers of being cornered, of being mauled. Nowhere was safe; nothing was sacred. I learned the art of hyper-vigilance, scanning my environment as if I were the gazelle in the Sahara. I was waiting, watching for the lion's attack. I knew no peace.

My young nervous system was on high alert every waking moment I was home. For two years, we played this game of hunter and prey until one day I broke. I couldn't hold the secret any longer. Standing by our car, in full display for the neighbors, I knew I had to tell my mother.

Frustrated by the heat, in a huff, she asked, "What's wrong? Why are you crying?"

Timidly, I said, "Dad has been doing some bad things, and I'm afraid you're going to be mad at me if I tell you."

Her eyes opened wide in shock. She stammered. "What has he done?"

While looking down, kicking the dirt with my sneaker, I mumbled, "He's been touching me and saying things that are sexual and gross. He asks me things that I don't want to talk about. About sex, if I have a boyfriend, and he touches himself while he's talking to me."

She asked me a few other questions, like when and where. Sheepishly, I answered each one. Fearing she wouldn't believe me, I cried my eyes out in our driveway while my guts spilled onto the gravel. I feared the worst.

Navigating the relationship with my mother was a maze of mind games. My stepfather's anger was explosive and volatile, so we knew what to expect. But my mother's attacks were methodical and calculated. Like a ninja in the night, you wouldn't know she had struck until after it was over. She felt superior by crushing your esteem and publicly shaming you anytime she felt you were getting positive attention. She often made promises that left you feeling like she had your back, only to realize she was playing you all along. So, I didn't give this situation much chance of being a successful mother-daughter bonding moment. Surprisingly though, she believed me.

Preparing me for what was about to happen, we walked in together, ready for the confrontation. And just like she said, he denied it. They screamed and fought with each other for what felt like hours while I shrunk in the corner by the door. My only hope was that this would soon be over, we would leave, and I would never have to see him again. Silently, as if chanting to myself gave me superpowers to fight the bad guy, I repeated, *stay strong, stay strong, stay strong*. In my mind, this was an unfortunate means to an end. This meant the torment was over. This was my moment of freedom. But I would soon realize, freedom would not come this day.

Instead, we stayed; we never left. Not another word was spoken about that afternoon. No one apologized. No one owned up to anything. We just swept it under the carpet, where it festered and rotted.

My stepfather, being found out, grew bitter and angry. My mother, knowing she had sold us out, turned her hatred for him towards me. She punished me for being the truth-teller. I was the target for our family's shame. We had all kept this dirty secret bound and gagged in the closet. But I opened it up, shined the light, and we couldn't un-see it now. So I was the bad guy.

The energy that continuously poured over me was poisonous. My sensitive system could not navigate the amount of hatred and disdain that came towards me daily. I was not safe. There was no sanctuary for my tired soul. To protect myself, I would hide away in my room. When I would come out for dinner, my mom would stop everything and announce, "Oh, the princess has decided to join us. Aren't we lucky?" Embarrassed, I would eat in silence and then go back to my room. I was the butt of the joke and the target for all the wrongs that would never be righted. Everyone in my family hated me, and it was unbearable.

Now 16, the topography of my life was changing. I fell in love with a boy, and my mother was furious. She loathed this relationship because I was happy. And finding happiness was unacceptable because my love wasn't being showered onto her.

Forbidding me to date him, she'd often come to my school to ensure I wasn't sitting next to him in class. When I dug my heels in and continued to date him she decided to strike at me. One day, in a fitful rage, she said, "You're going to sleep in our bedroom, but I'm going to sleep on the sofa." It was an utter betrayal given my recent past with my stepfather. Feeling hopeless, exhausted, and all alone, I tried to take my life that night. I wanted out. I wanted it to be over. I woke up after taking a handful of pills, in pain and disappointed I was still there.

When I turned 18, I moved out on my own. I bottled up all the pain and focused on my newfound freedom. I moved a couple of times, dated a few people, and married a narcissist who would be my son's father. When that marriage ended, I wandered between despair and determination. I knew there had to be more to life, but my weariness was getting the better of me.

The following years were a never-ending cascade of emotional wounds and broken hearts. I would crave connection with others, only to push them away when they got too close for comfort. I wanted to open up to them, be vulnerable, and share my truest self. But I didn't know how. I trusted no one, least of all, myself. My nervous system developed into a network of alarms, sirens, and red flag detections that provided me an easy escape route anytime I felt threatened. I was stuck between desiring openness and fearing captivity. It was lonely, and I didn't know how to change it. My trauma molded me into the perfect robot, programmed only for survival.

My healing journey started in my mid-20s when I went looking for therapists, coaches, and mentors who could help give me some sort of roadmap to my life. About ten years later, I stumbled upon an article that mentioned the relationship between empaths and narcissists. My mind was blown! It was as if the author had followed me around my whole life. For the first time ever, I felt validated about what I experienced, from as early as seven years old, and that it was called something. Peace washed over me once I gave terminology to what I lived through. I felt I mattered because I was an empath. I wasn't crazy, I wasn't too sensitive, and I wasn't too much. It was the reason I felt everything. It was why I cried during commercials and felt people when they were in pain. It explained why I would get overwhelmed in large crowds and why I needed lots of alone time to re-center and recalibrate. So much made sense!

I learned about Narcissistic Personality Disorder and how a person with NPD (diagnosed or not) abuses their loved ones to control them. It talked about gaslighting and how the narcissist habitually minimizes their captive to feel superior in their own minds. When I came to know these terms and truly understood that this was my family and a few of my past relationships, everything shifted for me.

This path eventually led me to the world of trauma-conscious coaching, where I began to fully understand who I was and how I was shaped by my childhood experiences. The deeper I explored this new terrain, the more I learned sad truths. With every rock I looked under, a new level of trauma would unearth. I was both intrigued and afraid of what I would find out next, but I had to keep going. It was in a somatic webinar where my mentor said something that shook me to the bone. "Empaths aren't born as empaths. They are not naturally vigilant and ultra-independent. The things you call "gifts" are, in fact, trauma responses. Empaths are empaths because of trauma. They are not born; they are made." I froze. Shocked and resistant, I didn't want to accept that.

I had just found some semblance of identity, and now this guy was taking it away from me! Struggling with this new information but wanting to understand, I surrendered and sat with it. Spending a few days mulling it over, I journaled, meditated, and questioned everything. And then I felt it. Somewhere deep, in the recesses of my inner child wounds, I knew. My mentor was right. Although I was born sensitive to my surroundings, I was, in fact, shaped by the harshness of my environment.

I navigated my mother's manipulation when I just wanted to be loved, all while she was just trying to win the game. I sneaked through life to avoid my stepfather because if my presence alerted his attention, I would get attention I didn't want. I listened intently to the sound of someone's breathing for an early warning system. I watched for facial cues and body language to read the person's emotional and mental state. My ears perked at the rustling of feet in the other room. Were they coming towards me? Was I safe? My instincts sharpened to a supernatural level, and it was all because I had to stay safe in a household that was anything but.

Accepting this new awareness saddened me; it broke my heart. As an adult thinking back to the child that I was, I mourned for her innocence. I cried for her loss. The more I held her, the more I healed. As I showed up for her with compassion, she began to trust. The softer I was, the more validated my inner child felt. As if I was her spirit guide, I journeyed back to her time and time again and held the space for her to feel seen. I told her it wasn't her fault. I promised her I would be with her from now on and that I was sorry no one was there for her before. I recommitted to her that we would be stronger as we moved into our future together. My words began to heal her. She met my eyes with tears on her face, and she smiled in agreement. I knew she finally felt safe.

THE MEDICINE

I've learned throughout my journey with relational trauma that to fully be free of our childhood wounds, we must re-parent the part of us that didn't have a supportive parent. That part of us that is still wounded. The inner child that feels abandoned and had to figure out life on their own is still in there, holding that memory. Like a time capsule, to them the trauma is playing over and over even though we have moved on in age. And try as we may, these wounds will never heal just by willing ourselves to press on and forget.

The most important step in that healing process is to speak to them with a different voice. If we are to heal the trauma, we must use a different voice than the voice that caused the trauma to begin with. We can be so hard on ourselves to the point of re-traumatizing those past wounds. When we berate ourselves for not being perfect, or we beat ourselves up for mistakes we've made, we're doing nothing but carrying on the tradition that our past abusers started. And abuse will never heal what has been caused by abuse.

Our inner child craves connection and safety. They seek experiences that will allow play and joy. But when we're the ones hating ourselves for not living up to some ridiculous expectation, it's the inner child that feels the pain. We might be adults now and far from the experiences that harmed us, but if we are speaking to ourselves in the same manner that our caregivers did, we might as well be there again.

The power to shift what was done, to allow the past to unravel, takes one simple act. We must show up for ourselves in a way that we didn't experience when we were younger. We get to love our inner child and show compassion for their experience. Our tone must be soft with the overall intention to create a space where the inner child can be safe. Nothing else will shift these wounds. No amount of cheerleading, motivational statements, or spiritual affirmations will heal us from the past if we don't first show up and allow them the space to be seen and heard.

Sounds so simple, right? Because it is. So simple, in fact, we tend to over-complicate it because we think the work needs to be harder for it to have value. But sometimes, when dealing with children, simple is the best course of action.

Reparenting the Child:

1. Notice when you are having an adverse reaction to something in your life, but you are cognizant that it isn't what it seems. A great clue: your reaction to what is happening is bigger than what is warranted. This is the perfect indicator that your inner child has been activated and needs care and attention. It could be a literal experience, as your present experience is triggering a past event exactly in the same manner. Or it could be more energetic as in what is occurring didn't happen like that before, but it reminds you of that time.

2. Take a few moments to yourself, a few deep breaths, and notice where in the body you are reacting. Where is the tension? Where are you activated? Once you locate that area, place your hands on that part of your body in a nurturing way. This is showing up for yourself in a way that you may never have experienced.

3. When you feel ready, close your eyes and ask your inner wisdom, "Who does this belong to?" Your intention is to allow the space for the child that holds this wound to step forward. Take your time, open and soften your mind's eye, and simply allow the process.

4. Once you get a sense of which age is holding the trauma, slow down, be with them, and let them know they are safe. There's a reason they are wounded. You rushing in to rescue or fix them isn't going to help. Your intention here is to validate that what they are feeling is difficult, that it's okay for them to be upset. Use soft tones, supportive body language, and compassionate statements.

5. After some time, when you notice the constriction has relaxed (because the inner child is relaxed), recommit to doing better moving forward. Set new healthy goals. Practice changing the habit

that keeps triggering you. Develop more self-awareness around the situation that still hurts.

In the beginning, this process might feel a bit silly. But with some practice and a bit of time, eventually, the wounds you carry will soften and begin to trust that they are safe. I know this is a practice that will be a game-changer for your life; I have seen so many miracles show up in my own. So what I've done is created an instructional video, just for you, to walk you through the steps so that you can do this powerful work for yourself. And as an added bonus, I recorded a meditation to guide you gently to meet your inner child and create a space for them to be safe.

You can find both resources at https://morrighanlynne.com/themedicine.

I know for me, everything I have ever experienced has led me to this moment in time, to be with you, to share this moment, and to pass on this valuable nutrition. I truly know how powerful this work can be. My only hope is that it enriches your life as it has mine.

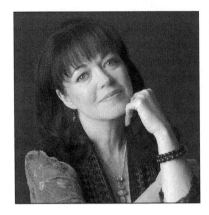

Morrighan Lynne is an Intuitive Transformational Life Coach, spiritual medium, psychic empath, clairvoyant, and author, having supported people from all over the globe. With a fiery gypsy soul and an eclectic approach to spirituality, she supports the ever-evolving human with compassion, straight-forwardness, and loving accountability.

Morrighan has received certifications through The Awakened School®, The Art of Feminine Presence®, and is a SafeSpace® Trauma Facilitator. Her style of coaching is intuitive and direct. Focusing on shadow work and trauma healing through somatic practices, she gets to the root of the problem and goes where many don't dare. A unique spiritual teacher, she has held 100's of workshops, retreats, classes, and galleries over her 16+ year career.

Having met her husband in Texas, Morrighan has put down roots in Boise, Idaho, with the love of her life and their two fur babies. She spends her downtime romping through the mountain forests with her husband, meditating, camping, paddle boarding, and hunting for mushrooms. She dabbles a bit in photography, loves to garden, and enjoys painting mandala art.

To see what she's up to these days, connect with Morrighan at https://morrighanlynne.com and get the latest news. Plus, be sure to take advantage of the free gift offered to you in her chapter by visiting https://morrighanlynne.com/themedicine.

CHAPTER 7

CRYSTAL ROSE
RAY HEALING

KARMIC CLEARING TO END SELF SABOTAGE
AND LIVE IN YOUR POWER

Asherah Allen, Lic. Ac., L.M.T.,
C.-S.C. Reiki Master Teacher Trainer

MY STORY

I am heading in to work to give a scheduled massage. The front desk informs me that another healer is using my room for a session, and she'll likely be exiting as I am arriving. I climb the stairs and *she* appears. Petite and fiercely angelic, her long blonde hair frames a beautiful, ageless face. It's the face of a priestess glowing incandescent with magick. She is a doppelganger of Kira, the Gelfing, from the movie *The Dark Crystal.* My jaw drops as our eyes meet. We are immediately locked in a soul gaze as we recognize each other from another lifetime. We forgo an introduction of names, and this seems normal given that we know each other so "well," as she states with an undeniable authority, "My guides are instructing me that you should sit down and I am to offer you healing."

Though dumbfounded, I comply willingly. Time stands still, and I feel between the worlds immediately, even though I was rushing about mere minutes ago. She stands behind me and begins to whisper. She pours out a gorgeous litany of words that I recognize as being anchored in the Egytian Mysteries and I feel a delicious tingling flow down my body and along my spine as she sends energy out of her hands into my auric field.

"It is complete", she states matter of factly.

"That felt so amazing. All the tingling down my head and spine. I feel great, thanks so much!" I stammer.

"It was nice to meet you!" she says smiling knowingly as she turns on her heel.

She seems to fly rather than walk down the stairs, and I am left still tongue-tied and somewhat amazed but vibrantly awake and alive. Truthfully, I feel a missing piece of my soul has returned.

I manage to get the massage table prepared in plenty of time to ground and center myself before my patient arrives. My eye catches one of her cards. It reads: 'Star of the Wayshower'. I feel I have just been touched by a walking, talking, adorably wise cosmic star. I feel that her visitation in my life was not by chance but mystically ordained. I am equally certain that I have just rediscovered a timeless friendship and that we will no doubt meet again.

Years pass and I move offices. As I am clearing out a junk drawer, I find her card and decide to call the number listed there.

"Hi Anahita! It's me Asherah." I say. "I don't expect you to remember, but we met a few years back at my office and I felt moved to call you."

"Oh I remember you! Yes! So good to hear from you. I've just moved back to the area, would you like to connect sometime?"

"Yes, I would like that very much." I respond.

We make a coffee date, and I am beyond excited, so a week later finds me at her condo at the agreed upon time.

She opens the door with a heart-melting "Hello friend!"

Once I am inside, she offers me water and a reading of tarot and oracle cards. As a reader myself, it is a joy to have someone read for me. It's clear she's very gifted: insightful, intuitive, and extremely wise. The reading is spot on and very helpful in guiding me toward the next steps on my path.

She begins to tell me her story. I meet her sons, and it is evident from the manner in which she interacts with them that motherhood for her is a divine calling. We revel in the love we both share for our children, and both give testimony as to how they are our best teachers and most clear mirrors.

She divulges that she is a stage four metastatic breast cancer survivor in full remission and was, at one point, years ago, given less than six months to live. I ask her how on earth she healed herself. She describes a mixture of conventional cancer treatment protocols and her own channeled healing system, Crystal Rose Ray Healing. I am amazed! She affirms that without question, this healing modality of hers has played a large role in saving her life. I recount to her the brief moment I experienced it when she shared it with me years ago and that I would love to learn the system too.

We are both very busy as working moms, but manage to maintain a strong friendship. She is consummately there for me and I for her. She forms a class to teach Crystal Rose Ray Healing, and a few months later I find myself in class with two other incredible women. Together, we dive into the mystery of her healing tradition. Anahita confides in me that she is on the spectrum, and she feels this plays a part in her ability to download and speak astounding amounts of information in regards to her healing work. I fall in love with her use of words and phrasing and am struck at how she owns her neuro-divergence. She admits readily to the fact that while often a blessing, it sometimes is a hindrance. She often asks me to restate things as she is impeccable at making sure she is correctly understanding all that is being communicated. I feel so respected and honored in my relationship with her.

I marvel as the bonds between myself and the other students deepen. I feel so much unity between the four of us, the deities we work with, the incantations, and the healing Rays known to this lineage. The lessons revolve around healing the Divine Feminine and Masculine within us all, the Ascended Masters, Isis, Sekhmet, sacred unions, twin flames, and karmic contracts. It is all so fascinating to me, and I am conscious of what a gift we all share in one another. We move through the training at a relaxed and steady pace for two years. Once the training is completed, we each walk out into the world ready to share this gift in our own unique ways.

The next few years are spent not only loving each other and deepening our friendship, but getting to know each other's children and feeling more and more like kin. Anahita is an adored friend, teacher, mystic sister and part of my soul family. We even start playing music together. Well, she plays her guitar like the badass she is while being wickedly patient with my faltering attempts to play bass. When I say badass I am not exaggerating. She has a picture of herself on her fridge in fishnet stockings, hair wild, ripping it up on the guitar and mike. She plays an old recording of her screaming "Pussy Power!" with a deep guttural growl that doesn't seem to be coming from her but from a large mythic lioness. She was a rock star turned healer, a Mama, a priestess. When we sing together it is pure magick. She has wild dreams of touring a radical musical ritual theatre show where I play bass and perform my belly dancing, and together we perform rituals for the crowd. I delight in her enthusiasm and scope of vision. We find ourselves constantly grounded into the reality of raising small children but keep our dreams, creativity, and play alive all the same.

Throughout our time together Anahita has a few scares with the cancer coming back but she always manages to keep it at bay. Through her healing system, she is able to conquer sugar consumption, which she feels grows her tumor in real time. She is able to break karmic patterns from unhealthy relationships that haunt her and steal the energy that she so desperately needs. She has managed to live a decade longer than doctors said was possible.

Then a day comes when I wake up and feel a rush of cold and nausea with an added intensity of the room spinning out of control. I yell, "Stop! Show me what is at the root of this!"

I see an image of Anahita floating in front of me and she looks very unwell. I immediately call her and she answers from the hospital. I am there within the hour, and as I walk in, I see a diminished, ashen version of the whip smart firecracker I have come to love so much. With darkened eyes and sunken cheeks, she says:

"I am not going to make it this time." I fall to the ground at her bedside and clutch her hand while doctors come in and out.

"I don't have much time", she mumbles.

"What can I do? How can I help?" I ask with exasperation.

My hospice volunteer years kick in and I find myself taking notes of what she wants for the care of her boys, her funeral services, making lists of action items to tend to her things, and then it strikes me- what will happen to her healing lineage? I leave that afternoon not wanting to tire her, but when I come back the next day I tell her I want to make certain her life's work continues even when she is gone. She gives me permission to teach what she has shown me, but encourages me to build on the teachings by walking with it in my own way. I am determined to honor this gift and legacy with as much devotion and enthusiasm as she has always shown me in our lifetimes-long friendship.

She spends months in and out of hospitals and care facilities, some of which are wretchedly, literally, haunted, Finally, Anahita is transferred to a calm and nourishing resting place. Soon I get the call from one of her earliest students that her hour is near. I rush to her side, knowing this is it. Her student reads a Quan Yin prayer for protection, and Anahita speaks about Sirius calling her home. It isn't a surprise to me that she is being called home to the star of Isis, she has always been otherworldly.

She passes with her sons and her family at her side, and then her friends are graciously allowed back into the room. We are very grateful, and we circle our hands around her angelic skin and bone, her remains. We feel the tremendous intensity of her spirit still in the room, and with tears streaming, we acknowledge how our lives have been deeply, deeply blessed by this incredible woman, this Mystic of the ages.

THE MEDICINE

Karma=When we realize something is wrong in our life and we need healing of it, we do well to acknowledge any lesson we've learned and then can ready ourselves to release it. If there is no identifiable lesson attached, but a pattern inflicted by systems of oppression or inheritance, then we can ask for that pattern and its effects to be healed and released as well. Karma is not a means of Creator to exact retribution but a vehicle for learning, soul growth, and healing.

DNA=DNA is the pathway Karma rides through all lifetimes in all time/space continuums and dimensions. DNA replicates karmic programs and trauma. It regulates the frequencies and energetics human etheric anatomy contains.

Self Point=The point from which the soul individuates from (while still containing the fractal concentrated energy of) the Goddess/Creatrix and becomes its own spiral iteration of awareness and own sovereign entity.

Allow yourself to come into a comfortable position. Maybe stretch or yawn before softening into relaxation. Let your mind wander while bringing yourself to a deep inner awareness. Your eyes may be open or closed, whatever feels right, true, and good to you. If you like you can tense your feet, and then relax them. Tense your calves and relax..tense your thighs.... relax....tense your buttocks... relax.... tense your back...relax...tense your shoulders... relax....tense your hands....relax.... tense your arms....relax... tense your neck....relax...tense your face....relax. Resting, releasing, letting go, I invite you to enjoy this meditative state for some time.

Imagine now if you will, an energetic cord descending from your sacrum anchoring you to the center of the Earth at its iron core. Feel yourself rooted deeply in Mother Earth. Imagine your energy intertwined into the star within the earth below to your soul's star above feeling the intermingling of the Cosmic realms and the deepest earthen energies coming into union in the center of your being, your spiritual heart.

State the following:

"I enlist the power of my Godsoul at the point at which it transmits and governs the laws of Karma, I ask you to heal, restore to wholeness, and fully align with Spirit, the double helix totality of my DNA."

When this process is complete you will feel a tingling sensation through the spine.

Now state,

"I ask for these healings through all levels and layers of DNA, the rational mind, the physical body and all its incarnations, all soul contracts, and spiritual evolutionary scales."

Once again, the process will be complete when you feel tingling through the spinal column.

Once you have received the clearing through all these levels, assume a stance with arms and legs outstretched and state the following:

"I now intend this healing to run through all Sex, Self, Passion, Pride, and Power Points and DNA nucleotides, to all points of Creation within and without."

Wait for the process to complete, knowing it is done when spinal tingling is felt.

Now you may intend the complete healing on all levels and layers of karma with relationships of those presently close to you whom you share your life with.

At this time I invite you to perform a recapitulation of your life taking inventory of any relationships, organizations, groups, affiliations, or ancestral inheritances that are unhealthy, harmful, abusive, or damaging. If a permanent ending to the shared ties with these souls and patterns is sought, you can now see, feel, imagine, or know the perfect tool to emerge that will cut away any cords of connection, trauma bonding, contracts, and karma you may still carry from these contacts, naming that person(s) or pattern(s) which you wish to sever from now. If it is your firm conviction and wish, you can through the powers of your High Self, command for this tool to now permanently and unalterably unwind, disentangle, and disunion from these bonds.

You can ask your Godsoul to release any character traits, complexes, self sabotage, behavioral patterns that do not serve and their respective complications.

Wait for the process to complete and know it is done when you feel the tingling up and down the Djed pillar of your spine.

Next rewire the circuitry with affirmations standing with arms and legs outstretched in a five pointed star, saying,

"I now stand in the light of my highest vision of myself, my passion, and my soul's purpose. I am now healed from all that stands between me and the most complete expression of my dreams. I now fully embody and embrace my most authentic self and every healthy way in which it expresses. With this act of healing I call my power and any and all soul fragments back to me from all times and places. Fill all that remains with the Love of the Holy Mother."

"I ask for this healing to run through all the levels of anatomy both physical and etheric, through all lifetimes and time/space continuums. I seal this healing with Divine bonds of Protection, with Perfect Love and Perfect Trust."

Again, wait for the process to complete and you will feel tingling throughout your spine.

When you receive the clearing through all the requests, place hands over your heart and state the following:

"I dedicate myself to Divine Love, I am ONE"

It is done.

Gently move your body, open your eyes, and arrive fully present, wildly free, and fully embodied in your power.

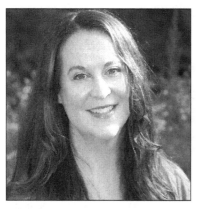

Asherah Allen is Certified Spiritual Counselor, Grief Specialist, and Master Healer. Her passion is being of service in helping people to live their most soul aligned, spiritually infused, radiantly healthy life. Asherah maintains a successful, private in-person and online healing arts practice. Her specialties include trauma and grief integration and pain management. She is a Licensed Acupuncturist, Chinese Herbalist, Licensed Massage Therapist, Certified Yoga Instructor, Meditation Teacher, and Reiki Master Teacher Trainer.

Asherah currently offers training in Crystal Rose Ray Healing and Grail Keeper Training as taught by Anahita.

As a Reverend, Asherah offers her services in performing marriage ceremonies, burial rites, baby blessings, sacred rituals, and house clearings. A natural intuitive and empath, she is a skilled tarot and oracle card reader.

Her notable institutions of study include a Masters Degree in Acupuncture and Oriental Medicine from New England School of Acupuncture, a Massage Certificate from Bancroft School of Massage

Therapy, and a Yoga Teacher Training Certification from Shri Kali Ashram, Goa India.

Her favorite pastimes include writing, playing music, and belly dancing.

She would like to acknowledge Anahita the founder of the Isis Sothis Star Mystery School and Crystal Rose Ray Healing Lineage, may she rest in power. Gratitude to Anahita's family, her Mother, Father, and sons for their love and support. Blessings of sisterhood in the Mysteries to Pamela Rosati and Carol Ohmart Behan. Asherah gives thanks to Justin Wellman and Melissa Brown for the great love shared by Anahita and for carrying this lineage forward.

Asherah offers her heartfelt thanks to her beloved husband and daughter for their unwavering love and support.

Her contribution is dedicated to all breast cancer survivors and to those who lost the battle.

To learn more about Asherah, get a free guided meditation audio link, or to book a service with her, please visit

http://awakenedhearthealingarts.com/resources/

www.awakenedhearthealingarts.com

CHAPTER 8

DARING TO DATE
THE DIVINE

CONSCIOUS DAILY BLESSINGS

Lulu Trevena, Artist, Quantum Healer, Soulful Living Coach,
Art of Feminine Presence® Licensed Teacher

"The divine plan is written with you in mind, sweet soul."

-Lulu Trevena

MY STORY

"Astonishing" was not a thought but a sensation that surged through me. I stepped through the plain door into the Indian Supermarket, Clothing and Craft store, in the main drag of the shopping district in Adelaide, Australia, and I was transported to another dimension. I was on my way home as an apprentice hairdresser, and there was something about this store on the corner of the main street that was beckoning me for a while. I was curious.

My body felt like it had ventured into a wonderland of exotic beauty; the colors were alive, sensual, perhaps even erotic; large ornate statues of animals and humans, melodic music, and the heady aroma of spices all lusciously cradled me. I felt inwardly and outwardly different. Expanded. Oddly, large and small simultaneously. I felt more. More me!

I was perplexed because only minutes before, I was just making my way home after a day's work! Mysteriously in the interior of the store, I was hit with a wild mix of spices and incense, as delicate, playful swirls of smoke and scent reached out, enfolding me, fixed where I stood. I felt in a state of bliss. Next, I was lifted out of my body, and I had a visceral memory and knowing of these sensations, aromas, fabrics, music, ornaments, and items of worship.

A memory of devotion and longing, but most of all, ecstatic bliss.

Time irrelevant.

I had had other out-of-body experiences at a young age, like when I was lying in a bath of warm water and staring at a candle perched on the opposite end of the bathtub, peaceful, serene, relaxed. The next moment, I, the consciousness part of myself, hovered near the ceiling, looking back at myself lying in the bath. I was in both places. I had numerous occurrences like this growing up. I learned how to naturally be still and connect. For most of my younger life, I was told I had "ants in my pants" because I was always active. I found this unwavering stillness, or perhaps it found me.

I remember hearing the words "Divine" and "Beloved." I have no idea how much time passed. I don't remember seeing anyone at all in the store. When I stepped back out onto the street into the fading day's light, I was transformed. I had gone through some metamorphosis. I felt intimate with the whole of myself at 17 years old.

This experienced stirred something awake. I would question my Catholic upbringing. I started going to Yoga classes, meditation, and Kirtan chanting workshops. I was seeking.

My inner drive was one of devotion and the longing of mooching up next to The Divine. Whatever you call the Creative Energy, God, The All of the All, Source, or The Divine, the journey is in finding an intimate rapport with that Being (Essence).

In some ways, I'm a rebel devotee. I want to know and experience on my own terms, not following any one rigid doctrine or path. In the past 35 years, I have never waned in my curiosity or my longing. I trained as a Yoga Teacher and taught Yoga and meditation for 15 years in Australia. During one particular class, I watched the students move into the postures, and throughout the room, I saw each person in a different part of the asana. It was like reading a Sanskrit text. Each person's body made up a character— four lines of students, 28 total. Unfortunately, I don't read Sanskrit, but the energy in the room was dynamic and effervescent.

I have had some deep experiences with mandalas, yantras, mudras, and chanting. My soul feels in resonance. I trust that these all support my journey. My trip to India in 2020, for the first time, was like a homecoming.

In 2015, I wrote an article for the Elephant Journal titled, *The Best Date of My Life*. One day, while meditating, I decided to go on a date with God/ The Divine. Here are some of the highlights.

- I showed up exactly as I was in that moment.
- I didn't feel the need to conceal any part of my natural appearance or enhance it.
- All my feelings were both relevant and irrelevant.
- All was valued, not dissected, made wrong, or denied.
- There was a deep acceptance of the myriad of emotions.
- We conversed intimately.
- Every word had relevance, reverence, and love aligned with it.
- Limiting beliefs, comparisons, judgments, and playing small were erased from my mind.
- I was listened to completely with focus and compassion.
- Nothing distracted The Divine from giving the gift of unwavering presence to me.
- Bliss was present and infused in each moment.
- Our hearts beat as one.

I realized that I was not dating God; I was dating myself. God was directing me always back to the greatest love of all: my own.

The last words spoken were, "My precious love, you are eternal, pure, and unrepeatable. Be only that which lights up your soul."

I humbly replied, "I will."

In my meditations, my self-committed dates with The Divine, I learn about my own self-communion, I receive wisdom about humanity, a breadth to compassion, and the depth of love woven through our existence. I surrender to the journey and welcome graciously the life that I have. I receive the blessings all around me.

I previously called myself a seeker, but much more often, I am the finder.

When I mooch up to The Divine in my meditation, it is a deepening, an exchange, a communion. A blessing.

You can see the full article here: https://www.elephantjournal.com/2015/04/the-best-date-of-my-life/

THE MEDICINE

"Blessed are they who see beautiful things
in humble places where other people see nothing."

– Camille Pissarro

We all know life can have challenges and be stressful. Taking small conscious steps gives us a good foundation for soulful living. I share here some practical, easy tools which, when consciously used daily, bring awareness, deepen our connection to a higher vibration, and cultivate wonder and delight. Many blessings can be spoken or repeated internally at any time and anywhere. You can invite blessings in and feel them somatically in your body.

We are the artist holding the paintbrush to the masterpiece of our lives. My hope for you when applying these is that they enrich your life experience, allow a deepening in the magnitude of your heart, and a connection to all life in its majesty.

Words have a potency and a vibration. We can use words to heal or harm. Many blessings have words that bring in a high vibration, clarity, and focus. If you wish to understand more about the power of words, please explore Dr. Masaru Emoto's work outlined in his book, *The Hidden Messages of Water*. It is an eye-opener. What we say has power.

When we wake up each morning, we have a chance to open to the blessings, big and small, that are all around us. None of us knows how long we have on earth, and that we wake on any given day is an indicator that we have another opportunity at living.

SEND BLESSINGS FORWARD

One of my first thoughts each day, as I flip my legs out of bed and let my feet touch the floor, is, *Thank You for the Blessings*. Starting your day this way sets the tone for openness and receptivity. You can also say it aloud.

When we do this, we're thanking life and creation itself. Choose words that feel generous and expansive, which are more empowering than groaning, turning your alarm off, and pulling the covers up. Please try it.

I believe we send gratitude, thanks, blessings, love, and good outcomes forward.

Often people write or speak their gratitude after they've received it. I use the power of intention by sending it forward. In other words, pave the road forward in the way and the direction you desire and then follow that path with faith and an open heart. I find words to be a healing balm, to connect, inspire, uplift, and offer possibility.

> *"Your own path you make with every step you take.*
> *That's why it's your path."*
>
> – Joseph Campbell

GREATEST GOOD

I have been using this blessing for over twenty years.

Divine, Beloved, please guide me with wisdom, faith, love, and goodness and place me in the environment and circumstances for the greatest good of all. Blessed Be.

I also say this after any frustrating encounter; it helps me be open to what I need to learn or integrate from any interaction.

LOVE IN YOUR SPACE

This is ideal when entering a room or a space. I do it each morning also as I enter each room in our home. Think of any doorway as an in-between place—you're moving from one space to another; the doorway is the threshold, a beginning point. I pause at the threshold, and touch both hands to my heart and say internally, *entering with Divine Love*, and then I release my hands, floating my palms forward in the direction I am entering. This can be a small gesture that no one needs to see if you do not want them to. Ideal in work environments, on transportation, or entering other peoples' homes.

SAVORING, FASCINATION, AND WONDER

This is a reminder to pause, be still, slow down, and soften your eyes. Connect with your breath, be fully present, and look around you. There is the old saying, "Stop, and smell the roses."

This practice is about savoring the moment, realizing it holds greatness and magic.

Keep curiosity as a companion, use the essence of fascination and wonder, connect and ignite these as your birthright to enjoying your life.

Start to choose these in any moment. Slow down. Pause. Soften.

Savor, embrace fascination and wonder.

I suggest doing this multiple times a day. Use your senses when you pause, bringing in subtle awareness from each of them. Our five bodily senses can bring us potently into the present when we deepen in the presence of them.

You may also enjoy my free resource using the senses: 5 Wonder Morning Rituals

https://livelifewithwonder.com/

EARTH APPRECIATION

Every day place your bare feet on the earth. In your own heart and mind, give appreciation for our planet, our home, to Mother Earth. Practice this with sincerity and deep honoring. Science and physics show us that electrical charges from the earth have positive effects on the body. This is a win/win, give and receive.

NOURISHMENT BLESSING

This blessing came from my training with Dru Yoga International. When my children were young, we spoke this each night at dinner, I continue to do so.

Dear Father, Divine Mother, Giver of Life,

The food that lies before me, so lovingly prepared,

I humbly offer to thee,

Source and Creator of all things.

I pray that in love, faith and truth,

I may use these simple fruits of the soil to better serve thee,

All mankind and to nourish the rising flame, our soul within.

FORGIVENESS - HO'OPONOPONO (make right, doubly right)

I have used this Hawaiian prayer for a decade, even as a daily mantra. It is ideal when you feel anguish or stuck, especially if you think you are right and the other person is wrong. This beautiful forgiveness prayer holds honor for all people. It restores connection, healing, and oneness. This helps to cleanse yourself of 'bad' feelings. Sit quietly, as in meditation and simply say the prayer:

I'm Sorry, Please Forgive Me, Thank You, I Love You.

These four simple phrases, used regularly, help develop love and self-esteem. I often say this before going to sleep most nights. Practice this prayer to feel and know its potency; you will be amazed. I encourage you to read more about this practice, to learn, and to appreciate the wisdom and richness behind this Hawaiian prayer.

HUMILITY, EMPATHY, AND COMPASSION (HEC)

These powerful three words can be generously added to any circumstance.

It is helpful not just to know the meaning but to embody the quality of each one. Read each one, then meditate on the feeling of each. Feel what each one feels like in your body, anchoring it in. Then call on any one of these powerful three in any situation as humble guides.

Humility - freedom from pride or arrogance, the quality or state of being humble

Empathy - the ability to understand and share the feelings of another

Compassion - a strong feeling of sympathy and sadness for other people's suffering or bad luck and a desire to help

BODY TEMPLE - LOVE IS HOLDING ME

This blessing was lovingly shared with me by Maya Luna. You can find her at www.deepfemininemysteryschool.com

Our body carries us through life. I like to think of my body as a temple, sacred and beautiful, and as we know all too often, we can think the opposite. As a woman, this blessing drops me deep into my innate divine feminine essence. I say this very slowly with reverence and love, pausing after each word. It brings delight, vitality, sensuality, acceptance, and love into my whole being. I often say it three times in a row or chant it for a period of time. I visualize a flower gently opening petal by petal when I chant this. Allow yourself to be immersed in this.

I am alive

I am here

Love is holding me

Right here

My body is the body of creation

My heart is the pulse of existence

My love is the ground of all things

INVITE WISDOM IN

This offering came from Dr. Christiane Northrup. As you go to bed tonight (or any night) consciously invite in the energy of someone living or deceased that you admire, someone who is/was a beacon of light, for peace and love to share their wisdom with you while you are asleep. Receive the blessings.

TUCK IN BLESSINGS OF APPRECIATION

At the end of the day, when going to bed, I take time to acknowledge something in myself that I feel proud of for that day. I tuck myself in with blessings of my own journey and growth. You can always find something each day.

Please practice these, weave them into your day and life, and feel the *blessings!*

> "*Give us the wisdom to teach our children to love, to respect and to be kind to one another that we may grow with peace in mind.*"

- Native American prayer

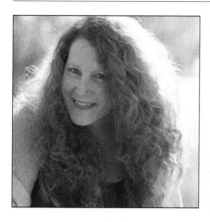

Lulu Trevena is an award-winning author of the stunning hardcover art and poetic prose book, *Soul Blessings*, winning the 2018 Silver Nautilus Book Award. She became a published author after age 55.

She is a Women's Workshop Leader, Quantum Healing Practitioner, Soulful Living Coach, Art of Feminine Presence® Licensed Teacher, speaker, artist, and mother. Lulu is passionate about shifting the societal narrative about women and age.

She is the creator of the card deck, "*Moments of Transformation*," and the hardcover journal, *Epiphany Journal and Playbook*.

Available at: www.livelifewithwonder.com/shop/

Lulu is the Founder and Creatrix of *Live Life with Wonder*. In 2020, she became a collaborative author in, *The Ultimate Guide to Self-Healing Volume 3*. She is also a collaborative author in Find Your Voice: Save Your Life.

In 2021 she was lead author of the international Amazon bestseller, *Wholehearted Wonder Women 50 Plus: Courage, Confidence & Creativity at Any Age*.

You can connect with Lulu at

Website: www.livelifewithwonder.com

Facebook: www.facebook.com/livelifewithwonder

Instagram: www.instagram.com/livelifewithwonder

Email: lulu@livelifewithwonder.com or lulu.trevena@gmail.com

For Women who want to explore, reconnect and reclaim her life with more wonder, take the Living with Wonder Quiz: https://livelifewithwonder.com/quiz/

CHAPTER 9

CHANTING IN THE AKASHIC RECORDS

ACCESSING POTENT HEALING AT A CELLULAR LEVEL

Laura Mazzotta, LCSW-R

MY STORY

Five years ago, I just wanted to be inspired. I needed momentum. Months earlier, I was bedridden after experiencing sepsis. There was so much damage to my physical body that I could hardly function, let alone think.

I was also depressed and anxious about what the future might hold. Lying in bed without focus, movement, or much of a spark, I had few options other than meditating. So, I meditated!

What I started to notice was how much better I felt the days I meditated. I thought *there must be something to this meditation stuff*, so I continued. I also investigated other alternative healing options, including energy and spiritual healing.

Several modalities started me on this path, but the most potent were Reiki (in which I'm now attuned as a Reiki Master), The Emotion Code (by Dr. Bradley Nelson), and The Akashic Records.

The Akashic Records blew me away the most because, when I was in this space, none of my symptoms were present. I had no pain, confusion, frustration, or discomfort. Also, when I would close The Akashic Records, I felt immensely energized! This was something I hadn't felt in a very long time.

The Records didn't quite make sense to me yet, but the results were speaking for themselves. So, what are The Akashic Records? I liken them to a spiritual library in the clouds, holding an infinite number of books, one for each soul sparked into existence. When you open your Akashic Record, you're taking the book of you off the shelf and accessing all the information about your soul, from its first spark through past lives, current life, and even into future lives.

The Akashic Records are a search engine for the soul: You can ask any question you'd like surrounding relationships, purpose, health, wealth, and the list goes on. This space is manned by angels, loved ones, guides, and ascended masters, truly making it the safest space in which to do healing work: You will never receive anything you're not ready to integrate when you're in your Akashic Record.

When you access The Records, you also tap into the deepest level of unconditional love for yourself, the world, and the universe. Your human presence becomes attuned to the high frequency of this space so, even if you don't ask any questions or do anything fancy, you will receive healing!

It took me some time to acclimate to The Akashic Records because I was so physically ill when I began. However, taking time to adjust is a good thing. You don't want to shift too quickly from a super low vibration to a super high one. That would be too jarring to your system. It takes the physical body more time to catch up with higher frequencies than our mind and emotions.

It's also deeply healing for human beings to have a regular practice of cultivating patience. I needed the space and opportunity to cultivate deeper patience for myself, not only to adequately explore The Akashic Records but also to gain greater insight into the inner workings of my physical body. Cultivating the patience for healing itself was a huge part of the process!

You can learn more about The Akashic Records and how to open them by clicking here:
https://www.theakashictherapist.com/about-the-akashic-records

Once I became well-versed in The Akashic Records (after much practice and guidance), I excavated the areas of most potent healing. The three main areas were 1) ancestral healing, 2) regression and inner child work, and 3) chanting.

Chanting is what this chapter will be discussing in greater detail. It's a skill you can cultivate on your own because it's straightforward, effective, and immensely powerful. Although being in The Records amplifies the experience, impact, and vibration, chanting can be done outside of The Akashic Records as well.

THE MEDICINE

The mechanism by which chanting is so effective is multilayered. First, and most important to understand, is sound healing at a physical level. Sound healing, especially when generated by your own body, is one of the best vibrational healing tools.

When sound is created, atoms and molecules in the air move rapidly and bounce off other molecules. The interactions between these atoms and molecules form different patterns. These patterns fall in line to create waves. Since energy is always moving, especially molecules in the air, these waves are very active.

The engaged sound waves travel into the vicinity of your physical body and activate your eardrum. Once your eardrum is vibrating, the fluid in the inner ear vibrates, sending a signal to the brain, which extends this frequency through the entire length of the body.

Cool, huh? This is how powerful sound, and what we listen to and speak, is to send the right signals to our physical experience. When you generate the sound, it becomes even more intimate because you are sourcing this incredibly healing vibration from within yourself. How empowering!

Setting an intention to create sound for the purpose of your own healing is deeply self-loving. As you open yourself as a vessel to the universe, willing to receive whatever is in your highest good, you fully allow and surrender. This releases you from all the holding-on in this world, allowing space for the most sacred, hidden medicine to come forward. That's the spiritual layer of chanting.

Cognitively, chanting allows us to bypass the mind in a very loving way. The words of the mantra themselves carry a vibration and hold compassionate healing power. Each of them creates a unique sound and meaning. This way, you can gently bypass the mind without engaging in direct conversation with it.

Also, when we chant in a language that is not our native tongue (e.g., Sanskrit), our ego cannot talk back with a retort of *that's not true* or *come on, seriously?*

Therefore, it's important not to sink into the actual meaning of the words you're chanting before you enter a chanting session. If your ego is attached to the meaning, it will get noisy and distract you! Talking back to your ego only engages it more, even if you're trying to set it straight.

Just allow yourself to get carried away by the cadence of the words you're chanting. The meaning will automatically affect you, and you will feel the emotional, physical, mental, and energetic shifts when you're not focused on the results.

Anytime you're doing energetic healing work, releasing your attachment to the outcome is key in receiving more efficient and effective results. When you fixate on what you're going to achieve from this experience, you're not allowing the vibrations of what you're doing to dominate the healing process.

It's important to surrender to the Divine wisdom of the universe to send energy where it is most needed for healing, rather than focusing on one area you would like relief. This surrender is when you literally feel your cells vibrating within you. You're releasing your physical body to this experience.

This release activates your parasympathetic nervous system (the relaxation response). Being in the parasympathetic state is vital to our health and wellness. It allows us to rest and digest with ease, giving our system a chance to breathe and relax, from our muscles to every integral system of the body. This naturally induces an emotional and physiological state of calm.

We are so used to the frantic pace of our world, but that isn't the state for otherworldly creation, prevention, and healing. It's the state of achievement, competition, limits, and burnout. We have access to infinite possibility when we are working with energy. It's always moving and regenerating. This regeneration is possible for our words, thoughts, emotions, and physical state!

In fact, each of your cells is surrounded by protective tissue made mostly of water. When we expose water to vibration, what happens? It creates a ripple effect in the water. When we expose our physical bodies, and thus the cells and their surrounding tissue, to sound vibrations, we create a ripple effect of movement and shifting.

When we fill our system with harsh sounds or critical words, our system will experience agitation at a microscopic level. This may not be consciously obvious to us in the moment, but it's a slow decline of our resilience in the background of our bodies. This consistent agitation will turn into inflammation and disease if we are not aware of its impact.

This information is not meant to scare you but to educate and empower you! The more you know about how these processes operate, the more dedicated you will be to making conscious choices in your environment (even if it's just the environment within).

The shifts that occur within chanting will occur how they're meant to, when we release the agenda of what we would like to happen and allow the energy to move into the space it's divinely guided. Open yourself to this magical process, and you will palpably feel the results, especially if you do it consistently.

How do you begin with chanting? Easy! I've condensed this into three simple steps:

1. Choose what you would like to clear from your field (e.g., anger, anxiety, pain, illness, judgment, doubt) and look up which Sanskrit mantra would be ideal for this intention (using an online search engine of your choice).

2. Find a free audio or video of this mantra (either online or in your music app) and write down the lyrics and phonetic spelling of each word.

3. Practice singing along with the audio/video until you find a cadence and feel more comfortable. Then chant the mantra repeatedly until you get it down! You don't have to memorize it, but you'll find a greater effect if you do. This is where time and patience come in! Take a deep breath and sink into the deep knowing that you will ultimately find your groove.

Also, quick tip: When you pause and hold your breath at the bottom of your exhale, you are cultivating patience for yourself! Add in this pause to make things easier.

Here is an example of the above three steps (although I always enter The Akashic Records first):

1. Choose what you would like to clear from your field: I would like to clear anxiety so I can feel a sense of peace (Hint: Adding "so I can," after what you'd like to clear will help you find a more specific and aligned mantra). After a quick internet search of "Sanskrit mantra for peace," you'll find Om Shanti Om as the best for inducing this state.

   In this example, I could have also searched for "Sanskrit mantra for anxiety."

2. You then search online for "Om Shanti Om video." Make sure to find one you enjoy in terms of cadence and melody. Then, read the lyrics in the description of the video. If they aren't there, do a separate search for "Om Shanti Om lyrics." Then jot down the lyrics, which are often repetitive. This one is:

   Om Shanti Om

   Om Shanti Om

   Om Shanti Om

   Then write them phonetically and practice speaking them word-by-word:

   Aum Shahn-tee Aum

   Aum Shahn-tee Aum

   Aum Shahn-tee Aum

3. Finally, when you feel ready, play the audio/video of this mantra, and begin chanting along with its cadence. You may feel a little rusty as you're learning and navigating this. Don't judge or criticize yourself! Remember, you will absolutely get it in your own time, and it will sink into your Being in the way it is meant.

   I encourage you to play with the speed, pitch, and volume of the chosen mantra so you can truly make it your own. Each mantra takes on a unique form as it interacts with our distinct energy. When you play with these specific qualities, you're enhancing the intimacy with which you chant.

Now that you've become a little smoother (and possibly even memorized this mantra) allow peace to permeate your Being. Close your eyes and allow your body to sway, your glands to sweat, and your voice to rise. Let your physical and emotional bodies move where they may, knowing you are powerfully shifting your energy in this very moment!

With your eyes still closed, note the shifts you are feeling. Take some time to journal if you'd like, or just sit in a meditative state for a few minutes to allow the energetic shift to integrate.

Integration time is just as important as the process itself! This was hard for me when I was sick because I just wanted to feel better right away. It's common to become impatient as human beings, wanting immediate relief and grabbing all the shiny-object opportunities that could make us feel better.

However, you will receive a much greater, long-lasting impact from your own healing when you deliberately set aside the time and space for the energy to settle in. You are healing at a cellular level! Do not take this lightly! The reorganization that needs to occur in the background requires energy and rest. In fact, you will do your body a huge favor by resting and drinking water as you adjust to this new modality.

After chanting and at least a few minutes of meditation, give yourself about one to two days for integration. See how you're feeling at that point and jump in again if you're called. You can choose a new mantra or use the same one. I like to use the same one until I feel like a mantra master!

Remember, you're programming your mind, body, and energy field. It's taken years to get to where you are, so there will be some rewiring to do within your nervous system. Give ample time for this to be integrated so you don't overwhelm the system with too much too soon.

Each time the area you intended to clear (e.g., anxiety, anger, doubt, etc.) arises during the day, repeat this mantra in your head or out loud. Allow a smile to form across your face, remembering the yummy vibration you got yourself to when you chose to chant earlier that day. This is how you maintain and sustain the vibrational shift from the chanting experience.

Finally, honor yourself for taking the time to do this! This level of healing does not just impact you. It impacts everyone you encounter, creating a ripple effect of healing for the planet!

As your energy field shifts, your energetic bubble overlaps with others' energetic bubbles, creating more of those waves previously mentioned. These waves enter wider and wider fields, so we can easily see how we are all connected!

Thank you for participating in this process. Thank you for picking up this book as your act of service to individual and collective healing! You are a rare gem on this path of spiritual and energetic expansion, with powerful wisdom and love to share.

To experience chanting first-hand, head over to the video tutorial I created for you to take you through this process: https://www.theakashictherapist.com/resources

Also, feel free to send any questions through the contact tab on my website. I would be happy to connect and assist you with honing this experience to your needs!

I'm sending you so much love!

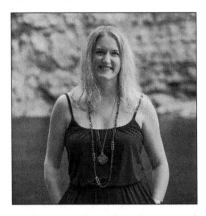

Laura Mazzotta, LCSW-R, is an expert therapist, Certified Akashic Records Practitioner, and Reiki Master with over 17 years of experience. Her mission is to guide spiritual entrepreneurs from deep, efficient, long-lasting healing to passionate 6-figure businesses, to serve the world from an even greater space of giving and service. Laura knows the most successful formula for limitless spiritual business expansion is potent, core-level healing combined with uniquely soul-aligned business strategy.

With extensive knowledge and skills in modalities such as EFT (tapping), Regression Therapy, Trauma Work, and intuitive development, Laura knows how to guide your healing journey in a unique, compassionate, and effective way.

During her recovery from a serious illness in 2016, Laura exhausted western medicine approaches and realized her deep passion for holistic methods, becoming an even greater advocate for personal development and transformation. Laura knows true healing occurs much more powerfully when all components (physical, mental, energetic, and spiritual) of a person's issue are addressed. She's here to guide her clients in all steps on that journey and empower them to share their natural gifts with the world!

Laura lives in New York with her husband of 20 years, three fabulous children, and one adorable golden retriever. She loves to be with family, create, read, and hike!

You can find Laura at www.theakashictherapist.com and join her free Facebook group: Room for Healing.

CHAPTER 10
SACRED VULNERABILITY

MOVING THROUGH FEAR
INTO COURAGE

Darby Ryon

*"I learned that courage is not the absence of fear,
but the triumph over it.
The brave man is not he who does not feel afraid,
but he who conquers that fear."*

~ Nelson Mandela

MY STORY

The smell of saltwater filled my nostrils as the sound of the crashing waves immersed me in my surroundings. I was chest-deep in the ocean, working my way back to shore. Each step was purposeful and intentional, knowing this area had sharp rocks and coral covering the seabed. Like the sway of a pendulum, the waves pushed me forward towards the sand while the undertow pulled me back towards the sea.

My daughter was walking a few feet in front of me with her puppy balancing on the paddleboard. The closer we got to the sand, the stronger the shore break grew. "I will carry your board in so you can carry Puppy," I said to her, thinking of the rocky conditions and wanting to protect her and my grand-puppy. Suddenly, I noticed the sound of the waves grew silent, and the pull of the undertow grew stronger. Knowing this meant a large wave was coming, I knew I had to move quickly to get the board so she could grab the puppy.

Pushing off the seabed, I leapt gracefully towards the paddleboard. The water kept me suspended as I flew in slow motion towards the board. In that moment, I realized I had thrown caution to the wind. But it was too late; I came down hard, feeling a sharp pain shooting into the ball of my right foot. I whimpered as I grabbed the board, steadying myself and getting my feet back under me. "Are you okay?" my daughter asked as she swung around. "I'm fine," I said, smiling through the pain, not wanting her to know that I had injured my foot on the sharp rocks. *I think I really hurt myself, that was so painful. But don't let her see your fear. Smile.*

Lifting the board under my arm, I gingerly walked towards the beach, with each step stinging my right foot. I stopped just shy of the water's edge, hesitating, looking at the sand, and wondering how badly my foot was cut, picturing sand grinding into the wound with every step. "What's wrong, Mom?" I heard her ask as she noticed I had stopped. My face twists into one of those "Oops, I did it again" smiles with teeth showing and eyebrows high. "What?" she asked again, "Did you hurt yourself?"

"I just bumped my foot on a rock or something. I'm fine; it's nothing." I responded. The fear slowly crept into my body, triggering the fight or flight mode. *Why am I hiding the fact that I hurt myself? What am I afraid of revealing?*

It was not about the cut; it was because I didn't want to show my vulnerability. It was my son-in-law's birthday beach party, and I was invited along with all of their friends. *Why do I have to be the one to get hurt? I wanted to be like everyone else, blending in, enjoying the water. It's bad enough that I am by far the oldest one here, and now I get injured?! I am the mother, the elder of the group. I must be the caregiver, the one who tends to others, not the one who receives care. I have to prove myself strong.*

I lift my foot out of the water just enough to see blood dripping out of it. I started to lose my balance and slammed my foot back into the water, just in time to save myself from toppling over with the paddleboard. "Let me help," my daughter insisted. "Naw, I've got it!" I exclaimed as I pulled up my big girl pants and marched up the sand to where the other paddleboards lay. Each step felt as though a knife was jabbing into my foot. I dropped the board in the sand and lifted my foot to see how much damage I had done. *Oh no, it's bad!*

"Well, that doesn't look good!" her voice came from behind me. "It's fine; it just has a little sand in it. I'll go back in the water to rinse it off," I said with an external smile and internal anguish, the sight of blood-soaked sand packed in a hole in my foot still lingering in my mind's eye. *Ugh, it is really deep. Don't let them see the pain, walk normally.*

I stood up straight and walked back into the water. Every muscle in my body, from my foot up to my neck, tightened when the cold, salty water seeped into the gash. I swished my foot through the water, trying to wash as much sand out as possible. Each swing through the water caused a burning sensation that made me hold my breath. *Keep smiling, keep smiling, keep smiling.*

"How can I help you, Mom?" she asked with concern in her voice. "Really, it's just a cut. I'll be fine." I responded, trying to minimize the severity of it. "But you could get me my flip-flops, so I don't have to walk across the sand again."

She brought me my flip-flops, and I slipped them on. Realizing my foot is throbbing and still caked with sand, I decided to go to my car to see if there is any way for me to clean or protect it. The farther away from the group I got, the more pronounced my hobble became. *I must get there without drawing attention to myself. Be strong.*

Pulling on the passenger side door handle, I swung myself onto the seat. The throb is growing stronger and the pain is pulsing through my entire foot now. There is a lump in my throat that is growing bigger by the second. *You can't cry. You mustn't cry. You have to show that you are a tough lady. Now get your act together. Quit being a baby!*

I was startled out of my thoughts when I heard, "Wow, that's a lot of blood!" My daughter had come over to check on me. Busted! I looked down and noticed the bed of my shoe had filled with blood. I heard "No big deal" come out of my mouth, but that isn't what my mind was saying. Not wanting her to think I was weak and needed help, I said, "Well, I should probably clean it up. Could you please get the jug of fresh water out of the back of my car?"

"We're going to need something to stop the bleeding too," she said as she looked around for something to use as a tourniquet. "I'm going to check to see what we have in our truck," she called while jogging towards her pickup.

"Oh wow, that's bad!" my son-in-law exclaimed as he came back from the truck with my daughter. *Oh great, now I'm the needy mother-in-law who is taking all of the attention at his birthday party. You've totally embarrassed yourself. You're never going to get invited anywhere. And now you can't participate in the beach activities. They will all think you are not the tough, adventurous type. They will think you are weak and boring.* My inner critic was having a field day with this one.

"We got this," he said with a big grin, holding out a roll of paper towels, duct tape, and a sock. "Thank you, I can do it," I stated, pulling the supplies from his hands. *You can take care of yourself. You don't need anyone.* "Are you sure? We want to help," he responded. *Don't take them away from their guests. You are tough; handle this yourself.* "You go back to your party; I will get this cleaned up and join you." I grinned, wondering to myself if they could hear my voice cracking or see my shoulders tense with the pride of independence.

My daughter stayed to help me clean and wrap it, but I shooed her away, telling her I would finish and come back to the party. Hesitantly, she went back to the beach to catch a few more waves.

Mustering courage, I hobbled back to my chair with the other party guests. Seeing my foot wrapped up as big as a football, they all said, "Oh my, are you okay?" Once again, I dug deep, pushing aside my pain and tears, and said, "It's just a little cut; I didn't want to get sand in it." *Don't cry, don't let them see you are weak and feeling vulnerable. Pretend you are brave and unaffected by this.*

I sat in my beach chair, watching the party guests enjoying all of the activities. Every so often, I would look longingly at the food table, too proud to ask someone to get me something and in too much pain to walk over myself. *Don't show any weakness, don't ask for help, you can eat when you get home.*

When it got to a point where my throbbing foot was consuming my every thought, I pleasantly said my goodbyes. "Do you want us to drive you home?" my daughter asked, walking me back to my car. "No, I'm fine. Thank you, though." *I hope I can drive with my foot wrapped and throbbing like a beating drum.* "I appreciate you, though," I said, hugging her tight.

I got in the car and drove away with tears running down my cheeks, more upset with myself for not asking for help and too proud to leave the party and properly clean the wound, wondering if all of my pretending really fooled anyone. *Why did I let myself get wrapped up in the mind talk? Nobody was judging me; I was just another guest at the party. Why do I always feel the need to be strong?*

I limped through the week, pretending it was fine. *Nobody else here goes to the doctor for a cut from the ocean bottom. You are worrying for nothing; stop being a hypochondriac.* The mind chatter continued, but it got to a point where I was not able to physically put pressure on my foot.

When we don't listen, the Universe will continue to gently remind us, getting louder and louder until it is fully in our face. Finally, I went to the doctor. By this point, I had a full-blown infection creeping up my leg.

There was no hiding it now; I had to stay out of the water and off my feet for at least a week. Once I came clean to my family and friends about how bad the cut actually was, they were all so kind and caring. Immediately, they started showing up with supplies for wound care, food, and offers to help grocery shop, run errands, or anything else I needed. They were there to support me, not judge me!

THE MEDICINE

We are told this world revolves around the survival of the fittest. Nobody wants to admit they are weak, as then they wouldn't be seen or heard. Admitting we are weak means we would be left off of that team, passed over for that promotion, rejected as a partner, or lose a friend. We believe we would lose respect if we demonstrate any weakness, so this creates a vulnerable situation for us. With that comes fear.

In actuality, it takes more courage to admit we are vulnerable than it does to fake strength. But to get past it, we must first admit that we are SOCIALLY vulnerable. When we desire to win acceptance from others, we are looking outside ourselves for worth and love. This desire overpowers our inner intelligence, our Self, the soul of our being.

"There is no fear for one whose mind is not filled with desires."

~ Buddha

Instead of letting our fear sabotage a situation, we should embrace the fear. Fear isn't our enemy. It is a part of us. Observe the vulnerability, accept the fear and release the attachment to the story it revolves around. These stories are born from the past, from assumptions, and from societal conditioning.

"What we are today comes from our thoughts of yesterday,
and our present thoughts build our life of tomorrow:
Our life is the creation of our mind."

~ Buddha

We have to allow our authentic Self to be seen. When we lean into the discomfort that fear creates, we embrace who we are at the core. Instead of pushing back and resisting fear, we can approach it with curiosity, having the courage to be vulnerable and take that risk. And when we express ourselves honestly, we become the mirror for others. We open our souls so others may see their own souls within ours.

To understand my behavior and my response to the fear felt in my situation, I had to ask myself some questions:

Where do worth and sufficiency originate?

I have been conditioned to believe that if I look, speak, think, and act like others want me to, I will win their acceptance, love, and approval. If I am seen as strong and independent, I will feel worthy. These are false and conditional promises, given and taken away on a whim. True worth arises from my authentic Self, my awareness of who I truly am, and my realization of the interconnectedness of everything. I am sufficient in my own Self.

How do I behave when I believe worth originates from the approval and acceptance of others?

I become an actor in a play, always living the life I believe others expect me to live. I act in ways I believe will cause others to bestow worth upon me. I portray a false image of myself, one that is acceptable to others. I am not honest, truthful, and open. It becomes a never-ending cycle, perpetually hidden behind a mask of fear. That fear is not being loved and accepted.

I am afraid of being judged as weak and insufficient, so I pretended to be something I wasn't. I was living a false persona. This is not who I am in my soul. I am trying to win their affection through false pretenses. I am putting on a mask to cover up the fear.

I was feeling insecure, that I was not worthy of connection. I am protecting myself from rejection, from being deemed as unworthy. I am protecting myself because I feel I am unlovable. I believe I am not enough.

How is this an opportunity for expansion?

I can become sensitive to those times I am being the actor, being inauthentic, and displaying a false persona. With this awareness, I can realize what I am doing. I do not need to "fix" anything, only discover and reveal my true Self. Then, I can speak my truth. I can live from the inside out. I can accept who I am and honor my thoughts and actions without judgment.

Love never arises from "without." Love is self-arising, sourced from my true Self. I have been conditioned to believe love can be given to me, that worth can be bestowed upon me. I was seeking love and worth from an external source, and that is a desire that can never be fulfilled. Love and worth are always internal revelations. When sourced from "without," love and worth are always conditional. When I reveal my true Self, I become love. I become sufficiency. Others can only support me in my revelation.

Our essence is pure love. Everything else is an illusion, a distraction from what truly is. We must surrender and release the attachment to the false stories, the created image, and distractions that keep us from pure love. Unconditional love comes from living in our authenticity. Love is only possible without fear.

When fear rises to the surface, and you are feeling vulnerable, ask yourself these questions:

1. **Where do worth and sufficiency originate?**

2. **How do I behave when I believe worth originates from the approval and acceptance of others?**

3. **How is this an opportunity for expansion?**

We fear rejection, being deemed unlovable, being seen as worthless. By allowing ourselves to be vulnerable and looking deeply at our fear, we can release the created persona, that false image of who we have created ourselves to be. We can relax and surrender to authenticity. To release the imposter and uncover the true soul is revealing pure love. Pure love has no attachments. It just is. It is total surrender that brings us to a space of pure presence. It isn't a gathering or collection of anything. It is the exact opposite. It is the releasing of everything we have gathered, stored, and become. It is nothingness, pure awareness, consciousness, the Self, and in that space, we are pure love. When there is no more searching, fixing, pretending, or expectations, then the only thing left is pure presence, pure love.

"Know that you are already liberated. You are never bound.
Thinking that you are bound is ignorance.
As the pure Self, you are never bound.
The true Self is eternally pure, unchanging,
immortal, never tainted by anything.
It is always peaceful."

~ Sri Swami Satchidananda

For more tools to help step into your Authenticity, connect with Darby at www.DarbyRyon.com.

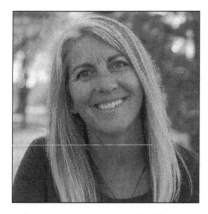

Darby Ryon is an adventurer who gathers friends and lessons along her journeys. Her wanderlust spirit takes her around the world and gets her into situations that will make you love deeper, cry harder and laugh louder. She helps others bring peace into their lives by bringing awareness to their authentic self. She guides people to be present with the disruptions and distractions that show up in our daily lives. Through this presence, Darby helps others connect with the Peace and Harmony we all have access to.

Darby became a spiritual explorer after her husband of 19 years died of brain cancer. She has had the honor of working closely with well-known spiritual leaders. Throughout her years of travel, Darby participated in the following courses: Life Force Energy Healing (Level 7), Past Life Regression Coach, Gateway Dreaming Coach, Clutter Clearing Coach, Tarot/Oracle Card reader, the Rites of the Munay-Ki (from Q'ero shamans of Peru), Red Lotus Mystery School and other spiritual programs. Add to that the technical and analytical abilities learned as a computer programmer and problem solver, her relationship-building abilities mastered as a Dale Carnegie instructor, her passion for exploration and curiosity as a teacher of children, and her appreciation of health and well-being as a professional Pilates trainer, and you have a well-rounded coach. Now she creates a safe space to help others discover what they need to serve their highest good.

Her passion is traveling the world to learn about other cultures and more deeply exploring the strong connection she feels to the indigenous. Her most recent devotion is to rescuing and rehabilitating injured sea turtles in Maui.

CHAPTER 11

INNER CHILD RETRIEVAL

HEAL THE PAST
AND AWAKEN YOUR MAGIC

Katy Jo Holton, Shamanic Healer

MY STORY

The sun peeked through the canopy of the trees revealing corners of the forest that otherwise would have been lost in shadow. I looked over at my cat, Blossom, who I named after a popular 80s TV show just a couple of years ago when I was five. Blossom hopped happily through the trillium perennials that were just beginning to get their spring buds. It was late morning, and the leaves made crunching sounds under my tiny feet as I made my way back into the woods. I walked past the circle of pines, beyond the mossy stump I carved my secrets into and plopped down on the soggy spring ground. Cradled by my favorite tree, I took a breath and closed my eyes. I knew there was magic here. With my back against my favorite tree and the sun warming my face, I listened. I realized the quietness of the woods has much to say when we are still and listen.

Years later, I found myself in a circle of fierce seekers and explorers from various walks of life, searching for answers and healing. I sat on a cushion readying myself for the ceremony. Deep inside me, I knew this space well. I surveyed the events of my life that brought me to this moment and gave myself some gratitude for listening to my heart even when I didn't know where it was taking me. I thought about the people I helped heal over the years and what I taught them. Today it was time to take some of my own medicine.

"My intention for this journey tonight is to become clear. I want clarity," I said as I looked across the circle of seekers. I had an inner knowing of what I was supposed to do with my life, but it always felt hazy; I couldn't quite see it. It was like swimming around in murky water, and the more I moved, the hazier it became.

"Ho!" The other seekers answered.

We waited until dark to begin our journey. As I settled in, I reminded myself, *the fear is the way.* Slowly, I quieted myself and began to observe my awareness. I scanned the edges of my consciousness and focused on my intention to find clarity. My mind would drift off onto other things. *I'm hungry,* I thought. Then I would catch myself and bring my attention back to the focus of the ceremony.

Why am I unclear? What am I not seeing? I wondered.

Way back in the corner of my awareness, I could sense her, my little one, the Katy Jo who sat cradled by her favorite tree. Her dirty blonde curls hung just above her shoulders. I couldn't quite tell what she was wearing. *Were those ruffles on her skirt?* She had a light within her, a magic and a purity that made me curious. I remember the gap in the two front teeth of her wide smile. That was long ago; little Katy Jo wasn't smiling now. She was very distant. I knew I had put her there, off in the darkest corner I could find, because her innocence scared me. I wanted her far away from me.

Later that night, my teacher inquired about my meeting her. I said, "I got in touch with my magical, innocent child archetype."

She said, "it's interesting that you call her an archetype."

I laughed. *That's how far away my little one was. I couldn't even call her by her name, Katy Jo. I could only refer to her as an archetype, some intellectual term that separated me from her and her from me.*

The next day passed, and the second night of ceremony commenced. Once again, I found myself part of a beautiful, loving space, ready to find the little one.

"My intention is to learn about innocence. Right now, I can only see how it is bad; I don't know if there is anything good that comes from innocence," I proclaimed to our circle of seekers.

"Ho!" The seekers said.

My journey began again. I settled in and reminded myself, *the fear is the way.* I thought some more about what innocence meant to me. To me, it meant naiveté, ignorance, unknowing, not to be taken seriously—words with negative connotations. Yet, I also knew I couldn't leave my little one off in the dark anymore.

I began to call her in; *where are you, little one?*

I could feel myself getting close to her; then I would retreat.

Closer again, and then a retreat. Closer and retreat.

What am I afraid of? I wondered. I quieted myself and became still. I reminded myself once more, *the fear is where the healing is.*

I looked in my consciousness once more. There she was in a floating, dark space, alone, quiet, scared, forgotten, dismissed.

I was so angry with her. *Why should I let you in? Why would I want you back? Look at what your innocence brought me!*

I showed her the time I was a child, alone for just a minute and that man put his fingers inside me. I showed her the time that boy kept touching me on the school bus. When I finally got the courage to ask for help, too embarrassed to say where the boy was touching me, the bus driver sent me back to my seat, ashamed and only to endure more of his assaults. I showed her the time my house was broken into when I learned that things could be taken from us in an instant. I showed her the time I was raped on the bathroom floor of my own home, where I thought I was safe.

This is what your innocence has brought me, little one! This is what you cause! It's your fault.

My body twitched and trembled as the sound of my pain pierced the air. Between the quiet tears, whaling arose from deep within my body. It went on for quite some time as I sat with the memories.

Then I became still. The scariest thing I could imagine was to let her come forward and speak. *The fear is the way.* It was time.

Why did you leave me here all alone? She asked. *Why did you put me here?* Her fists clenched in anger and her jaw tightened. She was fierce and direct and soft, all at the same time.

I asked, *what good are you?*

She was so angry and lonely. I could see how desperately she just wanted acknowledgment and love. When I finally quieted my body down and gave her my presence, she began to show me what I wanted to know. She began to answer my question.

She showed me walking through the northern woods of my youth, talking to the birds, speaking with the spirits, and with my favorite tree. She showed me waking up early on Saturday mornings to try to surprise my parents with breakfast. She showed me how the animals would come, wherever I was.

She showed me sitting on the back stoop of my quaint Georgia home at midnight, chain-smoking cigarettes. I had just gone through my first serious break-up, and my heart hurt so much from hurting someone else's heart. She showed me at the same moment bursting into laughter at the joy of the universe when I knew that even in our biggest pain, there is so much joy in this life.

Then she began to show me her magic. She showed me that innocence is a gift, that it was a mirror that showed us our truest nature. She showed me that innocence is being present with what is, without a story attached to it. She showed me that creativity comes from this place. She showed me pure joy. She showed me laughter. Then she showed me how to be empty and infinite. She showed me love.

I invited her out of the darkness, closer to me again.

I'm sorry for putting you there; I was trying to protect myself.

It was at that moment I realized all this time I thought I was protecting myself from being overtaken by someone else, and I realized I was protecting myself from being overtaken by myself. Slowly I began to see all of the perpetrators in my life as sacred teachers. Slowly I began to forgive them. I realized it was not my truest nature that left me vulnerable but abandoning myself that did.

I turned back to my little one. *Can you forgive me?* I asked.

She ran up and embraced me. *Thank you for keeping me safe,* she said. *Can I come home now?*

I moaned again. My body began to shake. It was one thing to turn and look at her. It was another to actually let her back in. At the base of my spine, I could feel energy building; I felt I might burst. I wept again and forged forward, opening my heart to let her in. The energy began to move up my spine in a giant rush of chills. But it was more than chills; it was spasms throughout my entire spine. My whole body was vibrating; I wasn't even sure if I could hold all that energy. I screamed some more but gave the energy permission to proceed. I was excited and frightened. My body quivered as joy ran through my veins. Her laughter began to echo in my being as I accepted her fully back in. Then I felt the light of her being rest in the center of my chest, and I whispered a quiet laugh. The little one and I began to play and dance together. She brought me through the woods; she pointed to her home in the stars, she showed me how she calls the animals. I created a space in my heart for her to stay. I nurtured her and watched her be the light that she is. Not a light for others, or me, or a light for a purpose, but because that was her nature.

I sat up and let her light reside in me and shine outwards.

Welcome home, little one. Welcome home.

A few weeks later, I began to notice the same energy return to my spine. It felt like magical chills that could barely be contained. This physical experience happened any time healing spirits showed up to work through me. It happened when I was healing myself. It happened when I was healing others. It happened when I was in the presence of beauty and joy. It happened when I was in the presence of deep truth. Since then, I have learned to use it as a tool to help me know when I am on the right path. It even reminded me sometimes to smile, for this life is truly beautiful. Sometimes I wondered, is that spirit moving through me, or is that me? I wondered if there is even a difference?

THE MEDICINE

Henri Matisse said, "The artist should look at life as he did when he was a child." When we are children, we are closest to our true nature. As our life unfolds, we have experiences that make us believe that we don't have control. To protect ourselves, we have an instinctive response to send part of our soul out of our body to prevent it from getting hurt. This self-defense mechanism keeps us safe for a while, but if we forget to call those parts of ourselves back in for too long, we might begin to experience problems like anxiety, depression, lack of confidence, or self-hatred. With part of us missing, we lose our balance and begin to walk in circles. When you find yourself in doubt, worry, stress, depression, or lack of clarity, there is a good chance that your inner little one is tugging at your sleeves, asking to be heard once again. Are you ready to listen?

If you'd like to learn how to retrieve your inner child, here are the steps to get you started. The next time you are in doubt, worry, stress, or negative thoughts:

1. Close your eyes and take a few slow breaths.

2. Ask yourself, *what part of me is triggered?*

3. Scan your thoughts to see if a memory comes up. Hint: it might not be a memory that seems directly related to your trigger; just go with the first thing that arises.

4. Visualize yourself from that time and name a few things you notice about yourself then.

5. Now ask yourself, what does that version of yourself need? Do they need to yell? Do they need comfort? Do they need to be heard?

6. Give them what they need.

7. When the time is right, embrace them and let them know you are here for them now.

8. Invite them back into your heart.

You can also visit my page: www.holtonhealingarts.com/innerchild, where you will find a free guide to help you with this exercise.

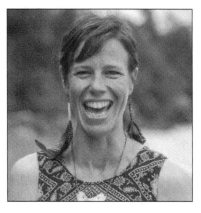

Katy Jo Holton, Shamanic Healer, Author, and owner of Holton Healing Arts Shaman School

Katy Jo Holton is a shamanic healer and the founder of Holton Healing Arts. She has 15 years of experience creating unique intuitive sessions for her clients. Her psychic skills guide you through connecting to your own inner knowing so you can heal your past, live with confidence, and integrate spiritual purpose with all aspects of your life.

Katy Jo trained with the Foundation for Shamanic Studies for four years while completing her MA in Transformational Leadership. Her training includes indigenous wisdom, non-native teaching, and direct experience. Her approach to Shamanic practice will allow you to step into your confidence in helping others and in navigating spiritual realms more powerfully. Through her Shaman School Program, you'll learn the necessary skills to heal yourself and assist others on their journey.

Katy Jo has walked many roads in her lifetime, making her a relatable leader who understands the balance of compassion and accountability. She currently lives in Anchorage, AK, where she teaches online Shaman School, does private healing work, and coaches healers. She also leads various workshops throughout the US. You can learn more about Shaman School at www.HoltonHealingArts.com

CHAPTER 12
SACRED REST

BE AT YOUR BEST BY DOING LESS

Kelly Myerson, MA, OTR

Quietly tiptoeing down the stairs, I attempt to avoid all the loud creaky steps. At my beloved Ninja coffee maker, I crack open a jar of freshly ground beans, pausing to smell their aroma before placing two scoops in the basket. Smiling, I reach up for my favorite mug with its red interior and the word "coffee" written all over it in many different languages. A clear *ding* indicates brewing has begun.

Moving down the hall, I enter my office and turn on my computer, navigating to the Calm App website. I choose one of my favorite songs and allow the music to begin to set the tone for my morning. Placing my hand on my heart, I take a deep breath.

What essential oil do I need this morning? I tune in to my body for how I'm feeling and to listen to what it needs. *I would like to feel hopeful.* I grab the roller bottle labeled "Hope" and roll it onto the interior of my forearms. Bergamot, vanilla, ylang-ylang, and frankincense waft into my nose. The calming effect is immediate.

Crossing the room, I pull out my meditation cushion and place it in the center of the room. I then remove my journal and a deck of oracle cards from the shelf and gently lay them on the floor next to the cushion.

From the kitchen sounds a quiet *ding*, indicating my coffee is ready. I pad down the hall to place the warm cup on the counter, add two scoops of my favorite creamer, and froth it.

Joy rises within me as the first sip lands on my tongue.

Ahhhhhh.

Savoring my first gulp of coffee, I return to my office. Each of my senses has been gently awakened.

Perching myself on my meditation cushion, I place my coffee cup on the floor next to the journal. I've made it! Here I am, ready to greet my day fully embodied, basking in simple joys, and returning to myself. Pressing my palms together at my heart, I close my eyes and sink into gratitude with a deep breath.

MY STORY

"I'm going to be late!" I wail as I dash around the kitchen, grabbing an apple, some crackers, and a granola bar and tossing them into my lunch bag. "I can't believe I overslept, again!"

I am so frustrated with myself. I'd meant to go to bed earlier last night. I'd meant to get up earlier this morning and make lunch, take a shower, and have time to rest before rushing out the door. Wishful thinking!

Quickly kissing my son on the top of his head and my husband on the cheek, I fly out the door, silently cursing myself under my breath. I slump into my car, begging it to start more quickly, and already dreading the lineup of buses I'll inevitably find myself stuck behind.

My anger rises with each passing minute, and it feels like every car is trying its best to slow me down more. "Just freaking go already! What is so hard about turning?"

When I finally reach the highway, it's backed up.

"Great, now I'm really going to be late!" I shout to no one in particular. I settle back into my seat and let out an exasperated sigh. This sucks. I hate traffic. I don't want to go to work and—*Shit, I left my coffee at home!*

My eyes well up with tears. Immediately, I hear a voice in my head:

What's wrong with you? Are you seriously going to cry about not having coffee?

I don't know who she is, but she makes the pit of my stomach fall. She's right; what's wrong with me? There are other people going through tough times, and here I am, ready to cry over a lack of caffeine and too much traffic.

Scenes like this one were my normal for many years. I identified myself as a "hot mess," not a morning person, always late, disorganized, unprepared, and NOT GOOD ENOUGH. I spent so many mornings this way, desperate to catch up. Other days were spent in bed with migraines, having crashed and burned. Worst of all, rest was something I got only when I was finally so overwhelmed and exhausted that my body gave me no other choice.

I looked on with envy at women who seemed to do, be, and have it all. They seemed to easily navigate their mornings, look great, find time to exercise and create glorious lunches. Next to them, I felt I'd never measure up.

I believed I was incapable of changing and overcoming obstacles to become effective, efficient, and effortless as a working mom. I celebrated my hot mess. I attached myself to the identity. And so it was.

Until it wasn't.

I began to crave something different. I felt a longing in my soul for peace, ease, and flow. Scrolling through Facebook and looking at those moms who seemed to have it all, I began to feel not just envy but a massive curiosity.

Curiosity was my in! I wondered, *how had they found happiness?* Then I wondered, *what makes me happy?* I scanned my memories for activities I'd once loved but no longer took time for. One idea stuck out: once, I was an avid reader. I devoured books relentlessly. Now, I really only read when I had time off.

But, I love reading books. I silently mourned.

My inner critic looked up at me from the corner of my mind. With one leg crossed over the other and a nail file in her hand, she glared at me. She didn't need to say a word. I felt her disdain and the smugness in her chuckle.

I decided to read more in spite of—no, maybe to *spite*—my inner critic! *Screw you; I'm going to find time to read! But how?*

I stood up a bit straighter as an idea popped into my head.

What if you listened to books on tape in the car?

"Brilliant!" I responded aloud.

Inner Critic rolled her eyes. *Remember, you're really bad at retaining what you hear. Do you really think you'll get anything out of listening to books in the car?*

Ignoring her for once, I logged onto Amazon to order a book and stumbled upon Audible. I signed up and snagged a copy of Eckart Tolle's *A New Earth*. It dawned on me that I had listened to this book on tape before, years ago. I remembered feeling capable of change and being present.

How many hours had I clocked in my car angrily commuting? In that tiny moment, I committed to change. I would insert joy into a time of my day that had become anything but joyful.

I woke up the next morning actually excited to drive to work. I giggled quietly to myself as I made my coffee. The concept of actually enjoying driving—in *traffic*—was ridiculous. But it also felt like a silent rebellion.

I paused as I placed the lid on my to-go cup. It had never occurred to me that the mundane could be fun. I mean, I recalled Oprah talking about something like that with Eckhart Tolle on her show. They had mused about how each step up a flight of stairs can be intentional and about becoming present with routine tasks.

Insert Inner-Critic-eye-roll here. I imagined her sitting there, sipping her coffee and letting out a big exasperated sigh.

Too bad!

Walking outside to my car, I found myself taking a deep breath and thinking, *Wow, the air is so fresh this morning.* Briefly closing my eyes, I tuned into the sounds of birds and distant cars humming on the highway. I liked the feeling of presence.

In that pause to breathe, I felt an awareness rising. I had a moment of peace and of being without doing. I smiled as I loaded my bag and lunch into the car. Once my phone was plugged in, I logged into Audible, and the soothing voice of Eckhart Tolle began to fill my car.

As I turned onto the highway entrance ramp ten minutes later, it occurred to me there had been few obstacles in getting here. *That's weird.*

Once on the highway, I found myself bracing for traffic and feeling annoyance rise into my stomach. I took a deep breath and silently reaffirmed myself; *It's okay; be here now.* My eyes settled upon the trees lining the road and the clouds on the horizon. They looked a bit brighter and more colorful than usual.

Pulling into work, I looked at the clock, surprised to find that I had arrived a few minutes early. I stayed in my car, closing my eyes to take in just a few more minutes of Eckhart's wisdom.

Since then, commuting has become joyful. Recently, I was talking to a friend on the phone during my commute. As I prepared to turn left onto the highway, the person in front of me was hesitating, though the light was green. I gently encouraged them, "Go ahead, friend. The light is green." My friend and I laughed at my silliness, but I felt so aligned with joy and inner peace that I could speak with strangers on the road as if we were friends.

What's truly amazing is how this one silent rebellion to find joy in the mundane became a mission to change my life. I began to prioritize joy and self-care. Sleep especially became a top priority, and with that, I discovered the magic in rest.

Like many moms, I initially approached the quarantine of 2020 with the intent to be amazing! I took pictures of my glorious homeschooling setup and reorganized work spaces. However, what made the biggest difference for my family was prioritizing sleep, nutrition, and rest.

Rest has become my superpower. In the evenings, I enjoy dinner with my family, clean and clear the dishes, and then walk away from work and technology. I set Do Not Disturb on my phone from 6 pm to 7 am daily. By 8 pm, my phone is silenced and plugged in across the room from my bed. I won't look at it until after my morning routine.

My day is bookended by sacred rest. It brings me greater peace and connection with my husband and son, and I have become much more efficient and effective in my work.

I choose my work hours and maintain boundaries around them. I decide which tasks align with my purpose *and* light me up. The others are either delegated to someone else or removed entirely from my schedule. By honing in on the essential few tasks rather than an overabundance of commitments, I devote roughly 12-14 of my 24 hours to serving my own well-being. My family receives the best of me. I exist in a state of overflow instead of overwhelm.

Filling your day with rest and sleep will first require a deep dive into determining what matters and what does not. Let's help you be at your best by doing less.

THE MEDICINE

Prioritizing rest takes both discipline and devotion. Each day, you will need to choose well-being. You'll also need to practice radical productivity and preparation. Those are life-giving magic too!

When I started to prioritize sleep, I considered the barriers preventing me from getting to bed, falling asleep, and staying asleep. Sometimes, I desperately craved time to myself in the evening after my son went to bed. I'd stand at an intersection forced upon a choice: either go to bed and get enough sleep or have time to myself for self-care and rest. That choice was bogus! Either I'm sleep deprived or self deprived! I know I'm not alone in this. We ask ourselves, *What should I sacrifice?*

But what if you didn't have to sacrifice? What if there was a way to have both great sleep *and* time for yourself? And what if you could also foster connection with your family? What if you could pursue your dreams and keep your home in order? You can!

Here are just a few practices I put into place. These are daily medicines—a recipe for well-being! You can find more tips here at https://beingwellwithkelly.com/sacredmedicineresources/.

BEGIN WITH JOY

Ask yourself, what lights me up? What do I enjoy so much that I lose track of time?

Create a list of your favorite activities—some inexpensive, some extravagant. Head over to my resource page for a free Joy List pdf.

Conversely, ask yourself, what do I *not* enjoy? Practice the discipline of saying, "No," unless it's a "Hell, yes!" Discontinue saying yes to please others.

Don't love a work or home task? Delegate it! There are no limits to delegating. Decide what your essential few tasks are—for home *and* work. Check out my resource page for some great books on this topic.

CULTIVATE YOUR CALENDAR

Infuse your life with joy and rest by taking control of your calendar.

Years ago, I learned about mind dumping and time blocking. First, dump your to-dos out of your head and rank them by order of importance. I use a form in Excel, which makes it super easy! You can find it on my resource page.

Then, block out family time, vacations, self-care, fun, and rest above all! There is power in putting rest in your schedule. Lastly, figure out your work and other appointments. Learn more about mind dumping and time blocking on my resource page.

USE TECHNOLOGY TO YOUR ADVANTAGE

Technology can be a time-suck, but when used effectively, it can support your well-being goals.

There are many settings and apps on your smartphone to help you set boundaries around technology use and your availability to others. Here are some of my favorites:

1. The Do Not Disturb setting. Set parameters for your availability by phone, text, and notifications.

2. The Calm App for relaxation, meditation, and music.

3. The Period Tracker App. It's not just for periods. You can save time by tracking all your medical concerns in one place.

4. Trello. It is a digital corkboard that allows you to create boards and move notes around. I use it to manage my business, budget, goals, opportunities, and more! Having one place to organize my whole life saves me plenty of time.

Finally, stop your technology use two to three hours before bed. Get high-quality rest *before* going to sleep.

Self-care is a choice, and by prioritizing fewer tasks and getting intentional with how you plan your 24 hours, you will find yourself at your best by doing less. Check out my resource page here for more ideas: https://beingwellwithkelly.com/sacredmedicineresources/

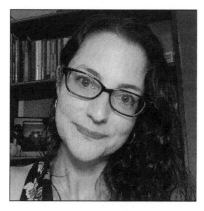

Kelly is an author, speaker, coach, and sleep expert who will cultivate space for you to emerge from stress and overwhelm to lead and savor the life of your dreams. As an occupational therapist, Kelly has over 20 years of experience specializing in sensory integration techniques. Her background in occupational therapy provides a unique perspective on development and the human condition. She helps overwhelmed working moms light up the world by taking them from burned out to radiating joy.

With a Master's degree in Strategic Communication and Leadership, she brings data-driven techniques leading to lasting change. Over the past 15 years, she has experience teaching topics including self-care, leadership development, outcome measurement, sensory processing related to anxiety, and sleep. Kelly is a holistic entrepreneur bringing a wealth of experience and fun science to inspire her clients. Most importantly, she'll get you the best night of sleep ever!

You can check out her three recent chapters, *Sacred Sleep: Cultivating the Best Sleep of Your Life* in the best-selling book, *The Ultimate Guide to Self-Healing, Volume 4, Courageous Self-care: Putting Myself First to Serve Others* in *Find Your Voice Save Your Life Volume 2*, and *Radical Self-care for Caregivers: Nourishing Yourself Through Grief and Loss* in *Sacred Death*. All available at https://beingwellwithkelly.com/books/.

For resources related to Kelly's healing journey and to connect with her, please visit https://www.beingwellwithkelly.com.

CHAPTER 13
HEALING SOUNDS

VIBRATIONS FOR YOUR BODY AND SOUL

Douglas Rarden, Nature Spirit Drums

*"Raising the vibration of the world,
one drum beat at a time"*

- Wayne Davidson, Nature Spirit Drums

OUR STORY

You never know how spirit might guide you during a meditation unless you do it.

It was during one of his daily meditations that Wayne was guided to begin birthing drums and rattles.

And Nature Spirit Drums was the result of his manifestation.

The fact that you're reading this book tells me that you have already begun to work in ways to raise your vibration, whether you're aware of it or not.

So good for you. The world needs you now more than ever.

Before I get started, I should preface this chapter by telling you that Wayne and I are partners in business and life. This year we'll celebrate thirty-seven years together, loving, learning, and growing.

To say that we were blessed to have found one another would be an understatement. It was 1984 when we first met, just before the beginning of the A.I.D.S. crisis. There are no words that can describe the grief and pain we experienced, as we lost the majority of our friends to this devastating disease. We were experiencing in our early thirties what most people go through in their seventies and eighties.

As you can imagine, we've become very connected to each other's thoughts and emotions through our years together and believe we are perfect partners when it comes to connecting intuitively through our work in sound and energy healing.

I grew up with a passion for music and singing, which I inherited from my mother. As a child, I remember her beautiful voice, as she would sing along with the radio or record player. She died from suicide at the young age of thirty-five. I was twelve.

But that's a story for another time.

Like Chiron, in Greek mythology, those who have healed from deep wounds, whether physical or emotional, become the healers of the world.

So when I heard crystal singing bowls for the first time during a sound bath, I knew we needed to add a set to our collection of instruments and healing tools. Of course, we weren't going to be satisfied with the notes A-G, covering each of the seven chakras. We had to have the sharps and flats too! Then came Tibetan healing bowls, two Native American flutes, gongs, chimes, Freenotes xylophones, body bells, crystal pyramids, and so on.

Yes, we're addicted, but don't you think it's a good addiction?

Every sound creates a different vibration and adds a new and beautiful layer to our sound immersion.

We were searching for Native American relics when we came across one of our favorite finds. We happened upon a hundred-plus-year-old Tibetan shaman's drum at a flea market near Taos, New Mexico. One can only imagine the shaman who played it before we acquired it. As the drum is played, you hear a rattle inside. Most likely from the bone fragments that were commonly used. It is truly magical!

Over the years, we attended numerous sound baths by many different practitioners. Each and everyone, creating their own unique vibratory experience. But it wasn't until about two years after Wayne began birthing drums that we facilitated our first sound immersion.

In discussing what we wanted to do differently from what we had experienced, Wayne said, " I want to incorporate the five elements, air, fire, water, earth, and ether, for our sound immersion." And so we did just that, by playing a plethora of instruments. And each one with unique healing properties, representing one of the elements.

We had the soulful sound vibration of the drums for those who needed grounding. The ethereal and sometimes otherworldly sounds of crystal bowls carry you up and out of your body. Powerful gongs that vibrate you to the core with their thunderous resonance. When played with the right tool, you'll hear the whale's song and be transported to the vast and boundless ocean. Then, there's the light, airy sound of chimes to still and quiet your mind.

One of the beautiful things about sound vibration is that those who are hearing impaired can also benefit from it. Whether you hear it or not, you'll feel it and receive all of the benefits.

We find that those with hearing deficiency are usually drawn to the larger, thicker hide drums, as they produce a deep and more resonant sound and vibration. Also, certain frequencies of the singing bowls may be uncomfortable for someone with a hearing aid, so we advise them to turn it off.

The first thing we do before any sound healing is tune into the person or persons present and ask our spirit guides to assist us in providing the type of sound and vibration needed to aid in their healing and raise their vibration.

Wayne walks among the clients playing a drum, rattle, or another handheld instrument. I accompany him with bowls, gongs, and other instruments that I'm intuitively guided to play. Occasionally, I chant or tone when my spirit guides nudge me to do so.

I bet if you think about it, you have many memories of experiencing a sound that touched your soul so deeply it brought you to tears. Or you can recall when the sound of a babbling brook, the song of a bird, or maybe a child's laughter brought you peace and joy.

Songs can send beautiful and powerful messages. And though you may not realize it at the time, those sounds and vibrations have a healing effect on both your body and soul.

The simple sounds in nature, the ones we're usually too busy to notice, are also profoundly healing.

It was right after our first event that we started receiving the feedback we hoped for. One particular client shared her experience, and it'll forever stay with me. I had previously done some hands-on energy work with her, so I was already familiar with her personal story.

She suffered a devastating event as a child. Her father had the intent of killing her mother and shot her in the face. Our client was not in the room but was in the house at the time of the shooting. Thankfully, her mother survived, but it resulted in partial blindness and some other physical challenges, and her father went to prison.

With her dad in prison, she became very close with her maternal grandfather.

She told us that while listening to the ocean drum, she envisioned walking the beach with her grandfather, who had passed a few years earlier. As she looked down at their embracing hands, she noticed that hers was that of a child's. A big smile appeared across her face as she shared her experience. She spoke of hearing the waves crashing along the beach, feeling the warm Gulf waters on her feet as the shining sun cast their shadows in the sand.

Our dearly departed are always looking for ways to reach out to us. Sound immersions can be one way for them to connect with us.

As she spoke of her experience, we knew she was beginning to heal from the loss of her beloved grandfather. The sound of our ocean drum brought about the experience, and we were blessed to have been a part of it.

On many occasions, we've been told that someone experienced an immense amount of energy coming from one of our ocean drums. Take a listen by clicking on this track, *Cries of the Sea*, from our second album, *SOUNDS of N.O.R.*

https://tinyurl.com/CriesOfTheSea

Others have told us about another instrument that monumentally affected them: the sound of a flute that stirred emotions or a bell that stimulated memories from years gone by.

The vibration of a Tibetan bowl can cause a reaction in the chakras that needs attention, bringing their body back into balance.

Many who have attended our sound immersions tell us that the experience brought them to see a rainbow of colors, each sound and vibration creating a different one. Some speak of geometric shapes and images as they soared through space and time. Others are moved to tears and don't know why, while some drift into a deep and restful sleep.

On occasion, someone has told us that a sound made them feel uncomfortable. If this happens, we tell them to focus on their breathing and allow the sound vibration to continue working on the areas calling for healing.

At a recent event, two guests lying next to each other felt as though they were floating above the sounds. They reached out to one another to ground themselves.

The magic of sound is that it can affect you emotionally plus have a profound healing effect on every cell in your body.

My first experience with light language happened while attending a sound bath. I was in a deep meditative state when I began to hear a foreign language spoken inside my head—a language not of this world. I understand it can be very different for everyone who experiences it. For me, the voices came very quickly, and it took all I had not to blurt it out as I felt the power behind it.

A couple of years later, while experiencing shamanic breathwork, it happened again, and this time I gave myself permission to repeat the language channeling through me. It was indeed a spiritual opening for me.

THE MEDICINE

I'm sharing how to break up and move energy in the body and how to clear a space of negative energy. You'll need a drum and a rattle.

If you already are the proud owner of a frame drum, this is a way to clear or move blocked energy.

If you don't have a drum, or your sweet little heart, desires another one, go to https://www.naturespiritdrums.com.

The first thing you'll want to do is, set an intention.

What is it that you want to accomplish?

Talk to your guides, ask them for assistance. Do you feel a strong connection to one of the ascended masters or archangels? Do you have an ancestor that you want to connect with to ask for guidance? If the person you're working on has a physical or emotional issue, consider asking for help from a spirit guide whose expertise would assist you.

We are all of one consciousness.

All you need to do is tap into all the help out there for you.

Now, you're all set to begin. It doesn't matter whether your client is standing, seated, or lying down. Start with a simple drum beat and use the same rhythm the entire time. The back of the drum should be towards the person you're working on so that they can feel the vibration of the drum.

Start at the feet and slowly work up their body, paying close attention to the sound of the drum. If you come to a spot out of balance or needs some additional healing work, you'll notice a change in the sound of the drum. It may be subtle, so listen closely. If this occurs, stay in that area and continue drumming until the sound changes back to the way it was. That's the signal that you have cleared the energy, and it's time to move on.

Don't give too much thought to what the issue might be. It could be a physical problem or an emotional one. Maybe some baggage carried over from a previous life. You don't have to know.

After you've reached the top of the head, turn your drum aiming the back towards the heavens. Keep drumming to send the energy into the ethers. Always thank your guides for their assistance.

We recommend that anyone receiving energy work of any kind should hydrate thoroughly afterward to help flush toxins from their system. Advise them to be gentle with themselves. It's all a process. REST!

Here's one way you can use your rattle:

Have you ever gone on a trip, and when you checked into your room, you could feel in your gut the energy wasn't quite right?

You may have felt a sensation that caused goosebumps up your arms or a queasy feeling in your stomach.

You don't know who stayed in the room before you. Of course, you have no clue what kind of morning the cleaning person was having or what negative energy they left in there for you to suck up.

It's a non-smoking room, so you can't burn your sage. Now grab that rattle you conveniently tucked into your luggage and clear the space. Remember, it's all about intention. Set your intention to remove the negative energy left in the room. Go from corner to corner, clockwise around the room, and shake that rattle.

Tune in to the sound as you shake it. Break up, transform and move all of that bad energy out into the ethers. You can also call on your guides to carry it away for you as well.

Wasn't that easy?

Hey, you're a sound healing practitioner!

With an open heart, some powerful intentions, and of course, a few beautifully and lovingly crafted instruments, anyone can heal with the magic of sound.

Just in case you haven't purchased your drum yet, here are a few things to keep in mind. Drums made from natural hides, like the ones Wayne makes, all have a unique sound, based on the type and thickness of the hide, as well as the size of the frame.

If your preference is a deeper sound, you might want to consider a drum made from a thicker hide such as moose. If you prefer a lighter sound, perhaps a deer hide would be more to your liking. Why not get both? You know, in case your mood changes.

Now that you own a drum or maybe two, you'll want to care for it in the manner that any sacred instrument deserves. Be sure to read the directions on how to care for your precious instrument at https://www.naturespiritdrums.com

Drum, Rattle, Sing, Chant, Dance, Heal, Love,
and Live the Ecstatic Life you were meant to!

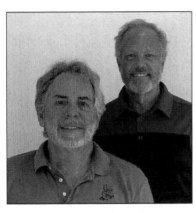

Wayne Davidson and **Douglas Rarden** founded Nature Spirit Drums in 2015. Both are shaman and sound healing practitioners. They're also reiki masters and master graduates of Deborah King's Life Force Energy Healing Course. They've studied numerous hands-on healing techniques and attended workshops and retreats with various shamans and teachers. In addition, they've experienced firewalks on three different occasions at The Gathering of The Shaman. Doug is also certified in Access Bars. Wayne's interest in nature and natural cures has taken him to study the healing benefits of native plants and herbs.

In 2018 they recorded their first of two albums, "SOUNDS, a Sacred Journey Through the Inner Cosmos." Within a year recorded their second album, 'SOUNDS of N.O.R Non-Ordinary Reality," and performed a track titled "Expansion" on Gulf Coast Meditation's "Awaken the Spirit Within." Their recordings are available on every digital platform worldwide. Their CD's are available at https://www.naturespiritdrums.com

They'll tell you, the thing that made the most significant difference in their lives is daily meditation and attribute this to their sobriety of ten years. Both are natives of Cincinnati, Ohio, and after spending 16 years on the S.W. coast of Florida, they felt guided to move to the Blue Ridge Mountains of North Georgia.

They facilitate sound immersions in the area and at their private residence, where they've created a labyrinth and medicine wheel to hold sacred ceremonies.

They're available for off-site bookings too.

Visit https://www.naturespiritdrums.com for drums, rattles, and upcoming events.

CHAPTER 14

MIRROR MIRROR

REVEALING THE BEAUTY WITHIN

Chelsea Lee Woudstra LMT, MTS, PAcP, Yogini

MY STORY

Dearest Reader,

This isn't the original story I planned for you. The magical medicinal tool is the same. My cherished friend Megan, who helped me edit this chapter, made some suggestions that changed how I wanted to deliver this gift.

"I feel like maybe you could add some things. Maybe more descriptors or analogies or something. I think that would possibly help it connect to more people," she said. "Not just ones who are struggling."

Her comments marinated with me for a bit in her lovely backyard that night, lit by the glow of the oil torches, and brimming with the sounds of laughter and conversations around us. It was the same message that woke me up at 2:30 am that night/morning and brought this out.

My original story was all about my loneliness, depression, anxiety, and unhealthy coping mechanisms that reared their ugly heads during quarantine; the plethora of demons I thought I'd slain over the many years of yoga, meditation, and inner and outer healing. It felt pretty relatable but read more like a journal entry. Megan was right. That may be many people's story too, but there's more. This reflective tool can help anyone at any stage on their path. We're all at different places on our journey toward the Self, however, it is coming to you here through the lens of my experience. Lisa Nichols, Louise Hay, and Tony Robbins are just a few of the world-renowned authors, teachers, and leaders who cite this tool as an aide on the road to "success." Their varied backgrounds begin to illustrate how impactful it can be for all different types of people.

So, while the main tool involves an actual mirror, this chapter is a brief collection of reminders that *everything* is a mirror of our inner world! Thank you for being on the continued trail to your greatest Self, dear reader. May these reflections inspire you on your way!

Much Love,

Chelsea Lee

"You're a *monster!*" She screamed at me from her terrified, red little face. That stopped me in my tracks. I couldn't believe what I'd done! My perfectly innocent five-year-old angel was clearly wrecked, scared stiff of her own mother. I had lost it again. My desire for control went off the damn rails completely, worse than ever before. I struck my child. It wasn't a tempered, well-deserved, conscious spanking, either. I felt the fire rising and burning wildly inside me, and then I heard the crack of skin on skin, felt the warmth in my palm, and saw the mark and fear on her face. She was right. I *was* a fucking monster!

I ran out of her room and down the steps to the bathroom. I locked myself in, as much for her own safety as my own. *Who the fuck was I?* I thought. *Some yogi! Some spiritual being! Some frickin peace-loving hippie!* My body was shaking and sobbing. I felt hot. My loathing for myself and my actions was beyond palpable. It was time to take a good long look at myself, both literally and figuratively. I had to confront this abusive monster. She had been growing within me for quite some time, feeding off all the resentments, triggers, past traumas, and negative inner dialogue and fueling the helplessness that turned to rage over the things I couldn't control. I wasn't listening to what she truly needed and wanted. What *I* truly needed and wanted.

What the hell is wrong with you? I asked myself as I studied my own flushed face of shame in the mirror. The truth was, I was sad, scared, overwhelmed, hurt, and disappointed in myself. Parenting is hard shit! That would be the understatement of the century, perhaps. All of my inner frustrations finally bubbled to the surface, and I snapped on this poor, helpless little girl, whom I loved more than anything in the world. It took me longer than I care to admit to process what happened and all I'd been thinking and feeling. I eventually calmed myself down. After bawling ugly-cry style in the mirror and thoroughly berating myself, I took some slow deep breaths. I forgave myself with as much forgiveness as I could muster at the time. I promised myself that I'd do better for Melody. I vowed I'd listen to and honor what I needed more, especially if that meant walking away sooner when the parent-child relationship began to boil my pot.

I went slowly back up the stairs to her room, where she remained. Shook.

"I'm so deeply sorry, Mel," I said sincerely. "Can you ever forgive me?"

She was still understandably keeping her distance. She simply glared at me.

"I love you so much, Melody. That was wrong of me to lose my temper like that. I get so angry when you don't listen to me, but how I behaved is never okay. You don't deserve that, no matter what. Not ever. Not from anyone, least of all the people you love and trust the most," I confessed. She softened. "I promise I'll never hit you ever again. I promise to deal with my own emotions better, especially my anger."

"I love you too, Mom. I forgive you. Please don't scare me or hurt me like that again," she requested in her sweet little voice.

"I promise." I fervently repeated.

We hugged and talked more. Our day improved as we laughed, played, and snuggled. I kept my promise and learned to listen to my inner voice more frequently, so the monster was able to stay softer, or when the softness was absent, I was able to be in tune when she needed some space sooner.

That blow-up was a big reflection of how my inner critic and all my inner dissatisfaction with myself and my life had compounded from my negative thoughts, beliefs, and stories. As I started doing more mirror work and regular gratitude journaling, I was able to see my life reflecting all the goodness back to me. Mel and I still had some struggles. It is, after all, life and parenting. Yet, all those dissatisfied areas of my life began to shift. So much of my anger began to dissipate, and I no longer took it out on her or anyone else. I now noticed it much more quickly and immediately apologized if I reacted from that place.

I made new choices from this new place of self-love and acceptance. Opportunities continuously flowed to me, and I seized them. I volunteered more. I worked more. I studied more. I made more time for my healthy friendships. All those things of which I'd been deficient, I chose to fill back up. All my gratitude and self-honoring practices were working! I made sure to do it every day, even on the hard days; in fact, *extra* on the hard days!

Everything I dreamed of just continued to manifest so easily. Work, play, and all of my relationships were better.

"Wow! You're an angel!"

"You're a lifesaver!"

"I feel so good! Thank you!"

"You're magic!"

"Thank you for helping me feel like myself again."

"You're so inspiring!"

"Mom, you're the best mom in the whole world!"

These were all reflections. These were the daily things clients, friends (and clearly that last one was Melody) said to me regularly. I'm not sharing this to boast, simply to demonstrate the power of these tools. The reflective clarity these practices bring forth is insanely profound! Such joyfully heart-warming mirroring of my transformed inner world and work, these words and messages were indicative of the major change to my inner monologue.

I got beautiful, recognized my self-sabotage, and spoke kindly to myself once more. Seriously. By throwing on a sassy outfit, some makeup, and talking myself up in the mirror, I began to heal. I was able to *see* mySelf again. We so often work from the inside out on this incredibly important task. When we're stuck and broken, and the inner tools aren't working, cleanse the vessel! Sweep out the cobwebs (or tweeze your eyebrows,) paint the walls (or your face,) and light a candle. See the inner light glowing brightly in your own eyes again! Beauty is an evolutionary part of existence, with a plethora of books written on this fact. *The Botany of Desire*, by Michael Pollan, is a prime and fascinating example of how and why plants have evolved for survival. Sunrises and sunsets, plants and flowers in bloom, stunning animals—their visual pleasure is a feast for the eyes and adds joy, comfort, and flavor to life. It also helps to perpetuate existence. Allow it. Embrace it. Yes, we are just as Divine, just as worthy of love, respect, and acceptance when we are naked-faced and in sweatpants, yet when we shine from the outside in and to the inside out, our own radiance becomes a blessing. We remind ourselves of our inherent loveliness. It is only a piece of who we are. It can be a powerfully transformative piece.

Honoring our beauty is grounding, creative, empowering, expressive, intuitive, and joyful! It was one of the many healing tools I used to shake myself back to life, and I've seen it work for so many others as well. As folks sit in my hair chair, share their deepest truths in front of a full-length mirror, I get to play Fairy Godmother. After they're done, they exclaim, "Oh! I feel like *myself* again!" I believe it is the marriage of the physical, emotional, and spiritual worlds that creates this transformation. By bringing my authentic self, seeing them and accepting them just as they are, and giving them a little physical boost or nudge, they can see themselves again! Realizing I was my own Fairy Godmother reactivated my magic. May you find her within you too, and send your cinderfoot self to the ball of life!

Now, it's way more simple to see when I'm internally off balance. Anytime we're triggered by what someone else says or does, it's an invitation to look within. The things we despise in others are almost always a reflection of something within us that we're ashamed of. Life, the Universe, Spirit, Energy, Source, God, the Psyche, whatever you name it, gives us the magnified version of our own inner disdain or unawareness. Reflections are both shadow work and light work. You can't really have one without the other. They are two sides of the same coin. The sun and the moon, we all need both. When we see something we don't like in ourselves, in life, or another, we have an opportunity for acceptance, compassion, and growth. It's exceptionally difficult to hate another human being when you've learned to understand that a part of them lives in you and vice versa.

When you know they are playing out their own human drama and healing their traumas on their own course, the judgments and resentments begin to dissolve. It's ongoing work! When we're brave enough to listen to our truth and softly shift it with love and intention for our own highest good and the good of all, that's where the magic happens. It's a balm to soothe all souls.

If you're repeatedly breaking things, having accidents, getting sick, in pain, attracting poor relationships, or struggling financially, something is amiss within. The other day, I was overly busy. I had too many errands, clients, and chores to do all in one day. In between shoveling a delicious meal mindlessly into my face hole, putting away the groceries, and serving my next client, the pesto slipped out of my cupboard from the top shelf, smashed onto my countertop, and shattered! An explosion of glass and bright green pesto was *everywhere*! I had mere minutes to clear it up before my next client. That was a mirror. It was a message to be present, to ground. *Give yourself more time and space to ground and be present. Enjoy life a little more—no need to get all wrapped up in all the to-dos. Breathe.* I gathered introspection from my own flustered energy creating such cause and effect.

When we ignore the reflections, messages, and synchronicities, they only get louder and more intense. *Wake up!* Our highest Self reminds us. It's usually easiest to learn to recognize these nudges early and regularly. There are loads of foods, workouts, doctors, medicines, healers, teachers, therapists, and books for guidance and healing. There are infinite actions to take to change our issues. We must start with the inner game first, though. We have to be courageous! We must be willing to listen and look inside, even if we are afraid that we might not like what we find. If I hadn't continued my inner journeying, I likely would have continued to harm myself and others. I would not have pursued it maliciously, but without the awareness or strength to not. You may not be as huge of a mess as I was. You may be barely a mess at all. In fact, I hope you are thriving already. If not, or if you're seeking to add in new sacred practices to enhance your life, read on. I know it can be frightening to travel into the deep unknown of the inner world. You can do it! We all can! You are a powerful being, capable of incredible things! I strongly believe in you. Please believe in yourself.

Melody and I made peace. We continue to make peace for ourselves and the world. May you continue to find peace, love, joy, acceptance, courage, and strength in yourself and the world as well, my friends.

THE MEDICINE

When you're in a funk, put on an outfit that makes you feel sexy!

Maybe throw on some special jewelry, or if you enjoy makeup for special occasions, doll up your face a bit.

Stand in front of the mirror. Full length is ideal, but work with what ya got.

Move your body and posture so that you feel strong and sassy.

Look deeply into your own eyes, and say your name out loud.

Say your name before each of the following statements.

Tell your Self five things you are proud of your Self for.

Tell your Self five things you forgive your Self for.

Tell your Self five things you *love* about your Self.

Say, "I am proud of you. I forgive you. I love you! You've got this, you strong, beautiful, brilliant badass!"

If it is uncomfortable, feels silly, or is challenging to come up with five things each time, lean in. Don't give up! You've got this!

Repeat this daily. Especially eye contact and words. Even if you don't feel like getting made up, shine your radiant love on your beautiful Self. You deserve it!

It may be challenging to come up with things to say at first. Here are a few examples if you get stuck.

(Your name), I am proud of you for surviving.

(Name), I am proud of you for continuing to grow.

(Name), I am proud of you for being yourself.

(Name), I am proud of you for trying new things.

(Name), I am proud of you for being brave.

(Name), I forgive you for being afraid.

(Name), I forgive you for being unkind to yourself/others.

(Name), I forgive you for playing small.

(Name), I forgive you for your moments of weakness.

(Name), I forgive you for the times you could have done better.

(Name), I love you for your courage.

(Name), I love your inner and outer style and beauty.

(Name), I love your kindness and generosity.

(Name), I love how you're always learning and growing.

(Name), I love you for saying yes to life!

I'm proud of you! I forgive you! I love you!

We've got this, you strong, beautiful, brilliant badass!

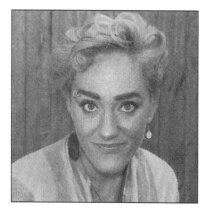

Chelsea Lee Woudstra is a Lovingly Transformative Force! Among other things, she's a Massage Therapist, Body Worker, Hair Artist, Yogini, Intuitive, Teacher, Speaker, Mentor, and Leader. She has been working in the wellness and beauty industry for over fifteen years and has a deep-rooted passion for helping others. Chelsea Lee practices a vast range of modalities, including Sound Therapy, Guided Meditation, Breathwork, Trapeze Yoga, Deep Tissue, Trigger Point Therapy, Myofascial Release Technique, Muscle Energy Technique, Energy Work, Acupuncture, and more.

She has trained at Aveda, and Vidal Sassoon Institutes in Florida, Michigan, and London, England. Work in the industry has taken her to Florida, Colorado, and Michigan. She is always looking for new ways to delve deeper into the work of creating a brighter self, and future for the universe.

Her life's mission is to reveal the inner beauty in each and every being she meets through authenticity and tailored practices. She aims to help bring others into their greatest alignment, working from the inside out and on all levels. She's happy to metaphorically (or literally) hold your hand and hold up the mirrors that you need to see.

Chelsea Lee also enjoys spending time in nature, and with her daughter, husband, and pets. Art, music, and self-discovery have been paramount in her life from day one!

She is available for local, national, and global speaking and virtual events, podcasts, and classes.

Connect with Chelsea Lee:

Abundance Salon and Spa Services LLC
NW Grand Rapids, MI 49504
(616)401-2603
hairbychelsea@gmail.com

On FB @ Abundance Salon & Spa Services
Join her Free Facebook Group, Align Divine
Instagram @chelsealeelight & @divinestylelight

CHAPTER 15

HEALING PREGNANCY LOSS

CELEBRATING THE SOUL'S JOURNEY

Susan Connor, PhD, ORDM, CRM

MY STORY

"We weren't able to find a heartbeat."

And with those words, my life changed forever.

I can only imagine what my face looked like because when she looked at me, the doctor's eyes welled with tears. I have forgotten her name if I ever knew it, but I will always be profoundly grateful for her compassion.

My husband was not in the room with me when we got the news, so I had to be the one to tell him. His face looked like mine must have.

I went home that evening from the emergency room with a deceased embryo still inside my body. I had not yet naturally miscarried, and it was around midnight on a Saturday, so there was no doctor available for a D&C.

I arrived home to my best friend watching my sleeping one-year-old, so I had to tell someone, yet again. I didn't want to tell anyone else. I was embarrassed. I had failed. A woman's body has one sacred purpose, and I had failed. I failed my baby; I failed my family. At that moment, I truly believed I had failed humankind with my inability to propagate the species. Never mind the sleeping one-year-old upstairs. Logic was nowhere near my brain.

Miraculously, I slept. I had two dreams that evening. In the first dream was a beautiful purple midnight sky. It was summer, and I could hear cicadas and smell honeysuckle. And then I smelled decay, and I realized I was in a cemetery, the kind with above-ground tombs that you see close to sea level. I walked deeper and deeper into the cemetery until I realized that my own body was a sarcophagus. I was frozen in place, and my only role was to house the dead. I woke in a cold sweat.

Later that night, I dreamed of my son, the one whom I would never birth or hold or nurse, but who nevertheless was still my son. I can see him from that dream space in my mind's eye today, a full fifteen years after that loss. He had a full head of curly brown hair, and he was not yet fully developed, although he smiled at me with a Gerber baby's smile. Our umbilical cord was still attached to him. A doctor in a white coat whose face I could not see came, and then my son was gone.

I learned later that between one in five or one in three pregnancies end in miscarriage—one in three. And yet we leave those women to mourn in shame and silence, or worse yet, not mourn at all.

If you are reading this chapter, you are likely one of the one-in-three. And you have likely read and studied and agonized over the physical reasons for miscarriage. Sometimes there is a chromosomal abnormality. Sometimes there is a health issue with the mother's body. Sometimes there is physical trauma. Sometimes nobody fucking knows.

In our case, we knew at about 12 weeks of pregnancy that there was a potential chromosome problem. An ultrasound revealed a thickened nuchal fold, which is a measurement of the fetus that can be an early indicator of one or more genetic issues. We were referred for an amniocentesis at 20 weeks, but we never got there. I started to bleed about a week after the ultrasound, and I lost my son.

I spent the years after my miscarriage wondering why my body failed and how I could have done different / more / better to bring that child into the world. I spent those years in shame and self-blame, and never once did my thoughts turn to the other soul involved in that equation—the soul of my baby.

Let me be clear, I passionately embrace science, and I am grateful for all of the knowledge it brings us and the health advances it has shown us. I take antibiotics when I'm sick, and my family is all vaxxed up. I understand that bodies enter the earth plane and leave it, and as often as not, there is a reasonable, scientific explanation for *why*.

But as I advanced in my own spiritual awakening, that reasonable, scientific explanation was no longer enough. More than a decade after the fact, I still mourned my lost baby, and sometimes, although less often as the years passed, I shed real tears over my inability to bring him forth.

It was then that I started to explore the spiritual reasons for miscarriage. The most comforting explanation I read was from a rabbi counseling one of his congregation after she miscarried. In his estimation, souls enter the earth plane for a specific, soul-contracted reason. Sometimes those lives last for 100 years on earth. Sometimes that soul completes its mission simply as a spark of life that does not live outside its mother's womb. We are not privy to that soul's contract, nor are we meant to be. Regardless of the length of human time that a soul lives on earth, its spiritual wholeness is the same. The soul's energy is never lost; it simply exists in a dimension outside our own.

I ultimately encountered the soul of my lost son, although at first, I did not understand what I was experiencing. While I was raised in the Catholic church and although my spirituality evolved over my lifetime, until my late 30s I was still very much involved in the day-to-day of my life, unaware of or at least had never experienced a soul connection outside the physical body.

Then I almost lost my physical body. One regular day as a mom, my son and I were in a serious car accident. On a routine drive to pick up my first-grader, my four-year-old and I were hit from the side at full speed when a driver ran a red light. Our SUV rolled, and when we finally came to rest, we were literally upside down, still buckled in but suspended from the car roof, sweet tea in my hair and everything from my diaper bag tangled the detritus of a typical mom car. The smoke from the deployed airbags clouded my vision. My son was terrified but not badly injured, blessedly still in his five-point-harness car seat.

As my awareness shifted, I realized that the car doors were jammed shut, and we had no way out. Bystanders had started to congregate outside the car to ask if we were alright, to offer assistance. I can still see their faces. One face, in particular, stood out from the rest as he was a child. He was about five, with brown, curly hair, round glasses, and a black t-shirt with a yellow lightning bolt. He didn't have an adult with him, and he circled the car looking at both my son and me, mildly curious it seemed, but not scared or worried. I lost sight of him.

As the doors to the car couldn't open, a man finally shouted at me through the window whether I could kick through the sunroof and come out that way. Barefoot, the impact having knocked the flip-flops off my feet, in an adrenaline-fueled movement, I put my foot through the glass of that sunroof without even having to work hard. I unbuckled my upside-down son and handed him out through the opening, then followed myself. Re-birthed.

Time passed, as time does. My living children grew. My spiritual awareness began to expand, and I awakened to the understanding of life beyond this life, of existence beyond time and space, of souls without boundaries, without dependence on the physical body. When I would pray for my children, either at church or in privacy, I began to pray as often for my lost baby as I did for the two pulling on my shirt and not letting me go potty by myself.

His soul blossomed into my being to be equally present, equally my son, equally part of my experience as a mother. At first, I thought he was present as my spirit guide, and he may well be. Gradually, though, I grew to understand that the soul he watches over is his brother's, the one born a scant year after his loss, the one who could never have been physically born had he grown to full term, the one whose near-death experience he guarded so closely that I could see him. He is always with us.

While I would never presume to know the soul's journey of another woman's lost child, here is what I can offer without doubt or reservation. The child, or the children, who grew inside your womb—whether for one hour or one day or one month or three trimesters—those souls are always with you. That connection is never severed, eternally present.

I cannot dismiss the grief and the sadness at never having known your child in this world. The lost experience of the labor of love to deliver them whole into the world. The nourishment of their body through yours. The joy of watching them grow. But I can promise that the soul is there and will be there, always.

One of the difficulties in navigating this path from grief to soul connection is the lack of understanding and acceptance of the necessary process. We ritualize birth. We ritualize Baptism or welcoming into a faith community. We ritualize passage through life from birthdays to graduations to weddings and anniversaries. We even hold funerals for the dead who have passed from a physical body into a plane beyond.

What passes understanding is that we lack a ritual to collectively mourn the loss of a pregnancy that does not reach term and to collectively support the mother who will feel that loss more keenly. We tell her to take a week and her body will heal. We tell her to try again. We tell her she'll have another baby to replace that one. We offer her an anti-depressant and a glass of wine. We tell her she'll forget.

She won't. She shouldn't.

The grief over a miscarriage is not linear. My mother, who turns 80 this year, still grieves the child she lost more than 60 years ago. And while, like most forms of grief, it does ease over time, it can also return in the most unexpected times and places: Meeting a child with the same name you had given them, the milestone year of a cohort to which they would have belonged, the anniversary of their conception or passing.

THE MEDICINE

The medicine I can offer you is this: the medicine is in remembering, rekindling, and nurturing the sacred connection that you and this beautiful soul will forever hold.

This is a ritual and meditation that can be repeated as often as you need. Some women choose to include their partner, and others prefer to take this moment for themselves. Do what is right for you.

Choose a space where you will not be disturbed, and create a comfortable area for sitting comfortably or lying down.

All of your senses will be engaged. Some ideas for stimulating each sense:

Sight: Gently light the room with a dimmer switch or colored lightbulb. Choose a candle in a color that resonates with your connection with your baby. If no color resonates with you, choose a white or lighter colored candle that can burn for about an hour. Bring in anything that speaks to you: family heirlooms, mementos that you had chosen for your baby.

Sound: If music or background sounds are comforting to you, select a track that will last for an hour without interruption. Gentle sounds like flutes or other wind instruments can also invoke an airy sense of peace and calm.

Scent: If you have access to incense, you may burn black or white copal. Copal was used in central and South American indigenous cultures during labor and childbirth to ward off fear, grief, sadness, and envy for the mother and the child.

If this does not resonate, you can also steam essential oils in lavender to relax and calm, jasmine to ease and comfort, bergamot to refresh and uplift, or any scent that brings you peace.

Taste: Brew yourself a tea of allspice, blue or black cohosh, comfrey leaf, or any other herbal that brings forth strength.

Touch: All parts of your body should be supported. Your head should rest on something soft. Your arms should be slightly elevated, so you feel almost as though you are floating but utterly embraced. If you are lying down, you can rest a pillow under your knees to support your legs. Every part of you should feel safe and comfortable.

Remember always that these are just tools, so embrace what resonates with you and leave what does not. Your energy and connection with your baby's soul are the only two key ingredients. You and your child are the focus.

You may take several hours or even days to decide on the atmosphere that will be most healing for you. If you repeat the ritual, you may change different elements based on where you are in your grieving and healing journey. There is no wrong way—your heart will know.

When you have settled your atmosphere, now comes the time to focus on you, your soul's energy, and the energy of your baby's soul.

We invite Archangel Gabriel, the angel of annunciation, to watch over and guide us. We invite Mother Mary to watch over and guide us.

Take a deep breath and hold it. Release the breath and inhale again deeply.

Allow your heart to travel in time and space to the moment when your body was joined with another, when your body was poised as a sacred vessel ready to receive new life. It's perfectly fine if you don't consciously remember this moment or were unaware of when it happened. Some people remember the moment of conception, and others do not, and the conscious memory is not important. Let your heart remember even when your mind does not.

And in that moment of readiness, feel into the stillness. At this moment in time, there was no "you," there was no "him," there was only potential and openness. And here, into this openness simultaneously entered the essence of the divine feminine and the divine masculine, at a space and time uniquely guided for a new soul to enter the world. Take a moment to look at each of them separately. Take in the beauty of the divine feminine in her glory, with her strength and her softness. Gaze at the beauty of the divine masculine in his glory, with his strength and his softness.

Witness both as they encounter each other and take in the divine love of that moment before they are joined, as they recognize the spark of life that will enter the world as soon as they touch. Bring your hands to your womb space and take in the knowledge that it is your womb through which this life will enter. It is your womb that has been chosen as the joining place of the divine to create new life, uniquely and perfectly guided to your body and to your heart, as the caretaker of its essence. This moment chose you. This soul chose you. This soul will always choose you.

Allow your body to remember itself as the sacred container for this moment. Breathe deeply as your body remembers.

As the spirit of the divine masculine and the divine feminine come together inside your body, feel the heat of your hands over your womb, at the place of their joining, at the spark of all life. At this moment, you are not just that soul's mother, but you are the All-Mother. You are one with the Divine Feminine who holds the power of life within her. You are one with the Divine Masculine who protects that life.

Breathe deeply as you look into the soul of that newly created life, the soul that chose your body for this moment in its soul journey. Say hello to this beautiful soul and welcome it into the sacred water element of its first contact with the physical body. Welcome this soul to your womb. Welcome this soul into your body and into your heart. Listen for its connection.

You may see an embryonic form; you may see a baby; you may see a child. You may feel a flutter in your womb space; you may feel birth pangs. You may sense a voice or a touch. You may not feel simply quiet and stillness. Whatever you sense and feel is perfect, perfect for the connection of this soul to yours.

Welcome this connection without judgment, without fear. Simply witness it for the beauty it brings in this moment.

Thank this beautiful soul for choosing your body, your womb, to be its earthly home. Listen with your senses to the name that soul used for you: Mother, Momma, Mom. Embrace that honorific and hold it in your heart.

Listen with your sense for any messages that your child has for you. You may hear words; you may hear a song; you may feel a presence or smell a scent. You will know when you receive a message. Breathe deeply and remain in this soul connection for as long as you feel called.

This connection is what you will remember when you feel grief, which you will still feel. This connection is what will remain when the grief passes.

Breathe deeply into this connection, and imagine the hands of Mother Mary on your womb, over yours. Imagine the wings of Archangel Gabriel gently waving over your entire body, bringing cool air, relief from pain.

When you are ready, open your eyes slowly. Breathe normally, returning to your body and to the present moment.

Return to this practice or some part of it whenever you need. The comfort is always here for you.

Then journey on, powerful mother, with the peace of knowing the connection between your soul and your child's continues, never-ending.

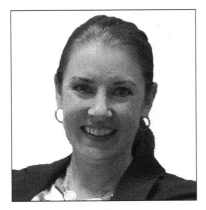

Susan Connor is the founder of Elle Qui Women's Healing, a practice dedicated to helping women find their purpose and heal from within. Elle Qui specializes in reiki healing, chakra balancing, and creating personal rituals that women can use to maintain harmony and balance in their lives.

As the mom of three, the stepmom of four, a daughter, and a partner, healing became a necessary function of life, which is what led Susan toward learning reiki and other forms of energy healing. Her practice includes crystal healing and aromatherapy, among other modalities.

In addition to Elle Qui, Susan also owns a customer relationship management consulting business and is part of the Women-Owned Business Network.

Susan is an ordained minister through the Universal Life Church, a certified reiki master, and she holds a master's degree and PhD from the University of North Texas.

CHAPTER 16

ANIMALS ARE THE MEDICINE

ACUPRESSURE TO RELIEVE ANXIETY AND STRESS FOR YOU AND YOUR ANIMAL

Josie Beug, DVM, CVA

MY STORY

One of the greatest obstacles in my life was obtaining admission and graduating from veterinary school. My intention was not to graduate and practice ordinary veterinary medicine utilizing pharmaceuticals and surgery. I was going to school so I could practice traditional healing, healing that used needles, herbs, and touch; healing that the modern medical world frowned upon.

At each step of my journey, an animal stepped up to give me just the nudge I needed to keep moving forward. Allow me to go back in time to how I decided on my path in the first place. It had to do with an animal, a dog, who communicated to me so emphatically, I heard him, loud and clear.

I graduated with a degree in biology and was trying to figure out what I would do with my life. When I moved to Portland, I got a job as a kennel technician in a local veterinary hospital, three bus transfers from my low-rent apartment. I jumped on the 4:30 am bus to make it to work by 6:30 am and have the kennels cleaned before the doctors arrived at 8 am. I scrubbed kennels and dog bowls and washed loads of laundry, so every dog received a clean blanket. I washed the dogs themselves, so they went home smelling nice and clean.

It was the middle of winter, just after the holidays, our busiest time for boarding dogs. An old Boxer had been boarding with us for several weeks. He was quiet and forlorn. This particular morning he looked even more depressed than usual. He was in a cage directly behind me as I stood at the raised bathtub, shampooing and washing the dogs who were being picked up that day.

As I was sudsing up a dog, I felt the Boxer's attention boring into my back, telling me something was very wrong. I kept looking back to check on him. He looked tired and had been getting picky about his food the last couple of days. When I got the chance, I pulled out his medical chart to take a look, something I rarely did. I was the kennel girl in the back, not the veterinarian. When I began flipping through the doctor's notes and lab results, I saw a report stating that a recent biopsy came back as an aggressive form of "neoplasia," a medical term meaning cancer.

If this dog had cancer and would die soon, why had it been sitting all alone in a boarding kennel for four weeks?

Something did not feel right. I ran the case by a referral veterinarian, who filled in once a week. As he read the report, a look of surprise crossed his face. I could tell he was thinking the same thing I was: the owners had not been notified, and the clinic was continuing to collect the boarding fees. We looked at each other, and he told me he was calling the owners immediately. They were there before the end of the day to pick the old boy up and take him home.

Soon after, at that same clinic, the veterinarian asked me to clean out a back room and throw some old boxes of stuff away. In one of the boxes of books, I found a treasure: *Dr. Pitcairn's Complete Guide to Natural Health for Dogs and Cats*. I took it home and discovered veterinarians practicing medicine a different way, using modalities I had experienced for my health care: nutrition, acupuncture, chiropractic, herbal medicine.

On the dedication page, it gave the name of a professional organization: the American Holistic Veterinary Medical Association (AHVMA). I called them immediately and asked the receptionist, "How do I become a holistic veterinarian?"

"First, you have to go to veterinary school," she replied. The next mountain I had to climb towered in front of me.

I was accepted into veterinary school several years later. I was one out of 80 students chosen from 600 applicants. The animal guides began making their appearance once again. On the very first day of class, I passed by the girl handing out the free dog food that I knew was filled with junk and spotted a Doberman laying on the floor with acupuncture needles sticking out all over her. Her owner, a third-year student, was the president of the school's student chapter of AHVMA. I knew I was home!

I fully realized that veterinary school was going to be a challenge. It was hard enough for a compliant student, but for one who went against the grain and had other ideas about healing, I knew I had to make friends in important places. I also knew I needed a secret weapon to help me out. That secret weapon was Reiki. Reiki allowed me to shield and treat myself and be able to treat and comfort animals, long-distance, across a room, without anyone having to know.

Animals that are sick and hospitalized, hooked up to fluids, recovering from painful surgeries, locked in cages away from their humans, were in more than just physical distress; they were in mental and emotional distress. I knew I would witness things that were going to be extremely hard on my sensitive, empathic nature.

Another canine teacher appeared on neurology rounds. He had just gone through a five-hour-long surgery, and I brought him into the ICU ward to monitor his recovery. The ward was packed full. Two emergency procedures were in process, the kennels were full of critically ill animals, and people were running everywhere. My patient's kennel was at floor level, so to get out of the way, I crawled inside the kennel with him and laid his head in my lap.

As I relaxed a little, I realized I had a dog's eye view of the hospital. I saw people rushing but from the knee down. I heard the echo of heartbeats as electronic rhythms, alarms from monitors going off, and people yelling from across the room, creating a cacophonous symphony of high anxiety rippling through the airwaves. I sat there with my patient, taking it all in, wondering what the animals were thinking.

Couldn't we do a better job and create an animal-friendly environment? How much was all this stress contributing to the dis-ease of our patients?

I sat there sending waves of Reiki across the ICU to the whimpering dog across the room, the yowling cat in the cage next door, and the little dog that was leaving his body as they performed CPR.

Oncology rounds brought a different lesson in healing. I stepped onto the oncology ward my first day, my doctor's coat ironed and crisp, my ears and eyes wide open, ready to glean as much information as possible. I always felt there were alternative ways of treating cancer beyond chemotherapy and radiation, but first, I had to learn this way.

My first assignment was to give a client the results of a nasal biopsy performed on their dog. I had never met the client, and the prognosis was very poor. The resident who assigned me to the case saw the uncomfortable look on my face and told me, "All you have to do is just go in and tell him."

All I had to do was tell this man his beloved dog was going to die, sooner rather than later.

One of the many trials of veterinary medical school is telling people really bad news about their beloved companions. We had no training in communication or counseling, but we did have on our doctor's coats and the stethoscope around our necks, our battle gear that was supposed to grant us confidence and status.

I stepped into the room, the little poodle cuddling up next to Dad, trying to squirm off the exam table. I introduced myself and told him we had received the results of the biopsy. I read out the words slowly: nasal adenocarcinoma. Before they had entirely left my mouth, the man's face blanched, turning white as a ghost. He half fell, leaning against the wall to the side of the exam table. I quickly stepped around expecting to have to break his fall. He caught himself and pulled himself back up to standing, his eyes aghast.

I grounded my energy down into the earth through my feet and told him to take a few deep breaths. I stood quietly by, holding space while he regained his composure. When he finally managed to catch his breath he looked over at me and said, "You probably are not going to believe me when I tell you this. A few months ago, I finished treatment and went into remission for nasal adenocarcinoma."

This was my initiation into the world of our animals taking on our suffering out of their great Bodhisattva-like compassion. I will never forget that man and his poodle and the love they had for one another. As difficult as it was, I am honored to have been the one to walk into that exam room that day.

Over the past 20 years, I have lost count of the times I gave a client a diagnosis for their pet and they reply, "I have just been diagnosed with that myself," or "I am taking those same medications." People feel guilty about "giving" it to their animal. I explain to them that their animal is mirroring the issue back to them out of their huge compassionate hearts. Our job is to support our animals on their journeys and be willing to see the patterns, heal, process, and make them whole again.

Another animal who touched me deeply and gave me the experience of mystical sight was an old grey mare. One way I got on good terms with the clinicians was to take a job in the clinical pathology lab and become the person they called to obtain emergency lab results in the middle of the night. This came along with its own set of risks, one of which was driving on ice and snow-covered streets at 2:00 am, at a moment's notice.

One particularly cold winter night, I was called into the lab. As I was preparing the blood sample, I could hear several voices echoing in the normally quiet barn. As I walked down to the barn to give the veterinarian the results, it had grown quiet, except for the sobs of someone crying, a little girl whispering through the sobbing, "I love you, I love you, I love you."

I turned the corner into the aisle between the horse stalls and saw the old grey mare, sway-backed, barely able to stand, and the little girl sitting cross-legged under her hanging head. I stepped back quietly and enveloped them in a bubble of gentle Reiki energy to allow them that sacred time together. The clinician walked up a few minutes later to administer the fatal injection. I continued to hold space for the girl and her horse.

On my way home on that cold, frosty night, I was sitting at a stoplight with no one else in sight. The air was so cold that ice particles were zig-zagging through the atmosphere. Something drew my attention up into the sky, and I saw her. I rubbed my eyes in disbelief, thinking maybe I was dreaming, and looked again. There was a white horse, young and beautiful, jumping across the night sky, mane and tail flowing against the wispy clouds. My heart filled with love and gratitude as the tears streamed down, nearly freezing on my cheeks.

THE MEDICINE

We all love our animals and want them to know how much we love them. The relationships we have with them are as intimate as those with our human loved ones, the animals often providing us with as much healing as we provide for them.

Connecting with them heart-to-heart, in a circular flow of loving energy, can allow us to communicate and exchange energy with them in a reciprocal manner, releasing and transmuting stagnant energy and emotions.

This technique is easy to learn and practice every day when you sit down to give your animal some love and rub their head. It is based on learning a few acupuncture points and a Taoist Internal Alchemy technique of sending and receiving energy.

Preparation: Sit up straight and take a few deep breaths. With every in-breath, feel yourself connect to the earth underneath you, growing roots down to the center of the earth. With every out-breath, feel the breath move upwards, out through the top of your head to your star chakra in the heavens above. Continue until you feel yourself anchored between heaven and earth.

After a few minutes, draw your attention to your heart center. With every breath, in and out, feel your heart center expand. Then feel the energy from your heart move down your arms into your hands until they feel tingly and warm. Now you are ready to lay your hands on your animal.

HEART HEALING:

Begin by bringing one hand between the front legs, onto your animal's sternum, midline on the chest. The acupuncture point here is named Conception Vessel (CV) 17, the Sea of Qi of the Chest. It corresponds to the heart chakra. Place your second hand directly opposite, on the animal's back over the shoulder blades. Feel the warmth of your heart energy flowing between your two hands until there is a bubble of warm rosy energy between your palms surrounding their chest. Stay relaxed, focusing on your breathing. Remain there as long as your animal allows.

CALMING TREATMENT:

Most animals like the top of their heads and their ears rubbed. One reason may be due to the acupuncture channels and points in that area. A great way to help them relax is to slowly stroke them, from the point between their eyebrows, an acupuncture point named Yin Tang, corresponding to the Third Eye chakra, all the way back along the bony ridge on the midline of their skulls, towards their ears.

There are several acupuncture points along that ridge that help to calm the animal's Shen, or spirit/mind, including Governing Vessel (GV) 20 and 21. GV-20 is also named Bai Hui, or 100 meetings. It is where the thousand-petaled lotus blooms forth when the crown chakra opens up. This is on the bony ridge, at the level of the front edge of the ears, and is excellent for calming the mind, relaxation, insomnia, even seizures. Some Taoist Masters say that it is the most important acupuncture point of the whole body and can treat all patterns of disharmony.

Once you learn these points, you can use them every time you pet their heads. I also like to rub flower essences or a few drops of diluted essential oils into them. Frankincense is wonderful for the head and heart points, to open to the flow of cosmic qi.

Animals are more sensitive to energy than humans. They will tell you when they want more, leaning into your hands or repositioning their bodies showing you the spot. They will also tell you when they have had enough. By being centered and grounded, it allows you to be more observant and aware of the signals they are sending you. Every time you honor their wishes and give them more or back off, you build trust and communication between the two of you. Listen to your animal and allow the energy to flow both ways between the two of you.

You can find more information about my work in the world and sign up for news and announcements at drjosies5elements.com and on Instagram @drjosiepetvet.

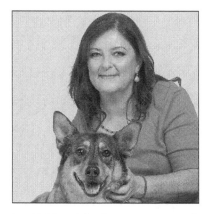

Dr. Josie Beug is a licensed veterinarian who specializes in Traditional Chinese Veterinary Medicine, among other healing modalities. She received her BA in Biology from the University of Colorado in 1989 with an emphasis in neurology. Before attending veterinary school, she worked for non-profit animal shelters for eight years. She earned her DVM degree from the University of Wisconsin School of Veterinary Medicine in 1998 with the intention of practicing integrative veterinary medicine. She was president of the student chapter of the American Holistic Veterinary Medical Association for three years and completed many externships with members of the Council of Elders of AHVMA. She has a thriving holistic house call practice in South Florida going on 20 plus years and is a lab instructor at The Chi University. Her articles have been published by Dogs Naturally Magazine.

She is a life-long student of the healing arts, from herbs to oils to energy to stones, integrating ancient knowledge with modern medicine to help her patients live longer, healthier, happier lives. She creates wild-crafted vibrational essences at Mollie & Me: Flowers + Stones + Herbs, https://mollie-and-me.com/. She has been on her own unique spiritual journey, guided by spiritual masters from Tibet to Peru and the thousands of animals that have crossed her path.

She can be found online at drjosies5elements.com, Facebook @josie.beug.dvm and on Instagram @drjosiepetvet. Sign up for her newsletter to receive information regarding her private online community, REVERENCE, dedicated to improving the relationship between humans and all other sentient beings on this beautiful planet we call Earth.

CHAPTER 17
THE DIVINITY WITHIN

AWAKENING THE HIDDEN INNER TRUTHS

Amber Dobkins

MY STORY

"This isn't about finding the right answer,
it's about the journey to inner guidance
that brings sacred truth."

Welcome to the meadows of sacred healing. The swaying trees, the flowing river, and the cool, grassy meadow all greet you with a warm hello. They are glad to accompany you as you awaken the hidden inner truths. These words came through me and onto a fresh piece of paper as I meditatively wrote in the woods of Southern Idaho. I let my hand glide across the paper while taking in all of my surroundings. I greeted the meadow of sacred healing with open arms, ready to be guided to deeper truths within myself. As I opened myself to the Divinity within, my heart began to feel warm and flutter within my chest. I was completely connected.

Feeling guided, I reached for a bottle of wine, popped open the cork, poured a glass, and gave it to the land in a ritual of gratitude. Connecting to everything helps me achieve balance and harmony with nature. I suddenly recalled science class teaching competition as the natural order of life.

I pondered this topic. What if competition is actually balance? Could balanced competition bring out the best in humanity? Balance isn't always peaceful. Sometimes balance is losing a job, being put on bed rest, or lockdown for a global pandemic. These seemingly devastating disasters can bring balance to a chaotic world. Let's take the global pandemic of 2020 as an example. The world was too busy, too loud, too chaotic. What did the lockdown do to balance that? It slowed us all down, quieted our lives, and brought some insight into the chaos. The lockdown was an opportunity to go deeper within ourselves. Many people found their passion, connected more with their families, dealt with deep emotions, and learned how to connect with the world in different ways. It's as if the Divine saw our unbalanced state and decided to throw a struggle at us to force us to find balance.

Struggles are there to connect us to our awareness and teach us balance. We can turn the struggle into a learning experience or even a pivotal moment of positive change. Many people seek answers to quickly ease their pain instead of being open to what the struggle has to teach them. When we connect to nature and seek awareness from within, we find the solutions we're looking for. Some solutions seem silly at first, however, they can bring massive change because we are being guided by our heart and not just our mind.

This isn't about finding the right answer; it's about the journey to inner guidance that brings sacred truth. Allowing yourself to explore new things guides you to your own truth and enhances your life no matter how the lesson comes to you.

I had to search for my truths and eventually save myself from my own constructs. I wasn't always open-minded enough to greet a meadow of sacred healing with open arms and ask for guidance. I was once a very closed-minded person, dying inside by not allowing myself to be the true me. Instead, I was desperately trying to become what I thought others wanted me to be.

I remember the first time I struggled with my identity.

"Look, honey, it's your new room," said my mom.

I was two years old, and for the first time, I had two bedrooms, one at my mom's and one at my dad's. The divorce made me question where I actually belonged. As time went on, I eventually had two separate sets of clothing, two separate sets of toys, and even two separate sets of siblings. Then came the separation of my last name—two separate last names. My name no longer tied me to one family unit; it now tied me to two separate families, with me being the only thing that connected them. My soul felt pulled in opposing directions and lost in the mix of two extremely different worlds.

When I started school, I was given the option to use my mother's or my father's last name. I always used only one last name, but I changed which one I used at times. My name choice was usually based on which parent I was living with during the school year. It became difficult for me to know who I truly was when I had two identities.

Eventually, I finished school and realized the adult world didn't care which name I preferred; instead, it demanded which name I used based on my legal documents. In some ways, this made life easier; in other ways, it made me feel like I could no longer choose my identity.

Shortly after becoming an adult, it didn't matter who I was because I was in love. Love didn't mind which last name I used since it would change when the handsome young man I was engaged to said, "I do." Our wedding day quickly approached. I remember the exact moment my name legally changed.

"Do you?" asked the minister.

My love responded, "I do."

The minister turned to me. "And do you?" He might as well have finished the sentence with, "take this man's last name?"

"I do," quickly flew from my mouth.

I always dreamed of one day feeling secure in a name and who I was. The day had finally come, and I was ecstatic about my new identity.

We had our first child prior to getting married and then, immediately after our wedding, rushed to have our second child. Our little ones were three years apart. After having our second child, I decided I couldn't bear to leave our children in the care of someone else. So I justified the financial savings of me staying home by making cheap, homemade meals, spending less on gas, and eliminating child care expenses. I officially became a stay-at-home mom, or as I liked to call it, a homemaker. I proudly placed that title on documents in the box labeled occupation. I immediately took my occupation seriously and looked up stay-at-home mom groups, found all the nearby parks, ordered at-home educational material, and set a strict schedule. Now I had all my ducks in a row—or so I thought.

I slowly looked around my home and saw the dishes overflowing in the sink, the laundry eyeballing me for attention, and heard my kids fighting in the other room. I looked at the time to see how much longer before my husband would be home. I could at least use some adult conversation while I tended to the demanding household chores. It was only 9 am. It would be another twelve hours before he would come home. Being a homemaker was harder than I anticipated.

My husband was working full-time and carried a full load of credits at the local university. On top of his insane schedule, he was also on the college bowling team, which required several weekend trips to compete all over the western United States. With competitions looming over him, he also had to fit in practice time and still study for his classes. When feeling lonely and overwhelmed, I tried to comfort myself with the thought that he only had two more years left in college.

Those two years turned into six before he received his Bachelor's degree. During those six years, my life felt like it was one big load of laundry that never ended. I repeated my long days of household duties, motherly obligation, and of course, my role as wife, day in and day out. It wasn't so much the repetition; it was the lack of connection and the constant loneliness that finally made me resentful of all the time we'd lost together. After my husband graduated college, things didn't change much. He was still gone all the time; it was just for social activities now instead of class. He worked for so long on his degree that he had to make up for all the playtime he missed over the years. I was happy for him but still felt extremely lonely.

Who am I? What am I meant to do here on earth? What am I doing wrong to deserve this emotional misery? These were the questions I pondered as tears slowly slid down my cheeks at night. I numbed the lump in my throat and clenched my pillow to quiet my sobs so my husband wouldn't know I was crying. I wanted to hide my face in my pillow forever. I didn't want to be seen, touched, needed, or forced to make another decision. It was all too painful. *Please, God, take me in my sleep*, was my silent prayer. Even though I was religious at the time, I never heard God speak back; I was always left in silence, which brought more frustration and eventually anger. I was angry at God, my husband, my kids, but even more so at myself. How did I allow myself to get to this point? I was dead inside. My soul ached, and I didn't know how to soothe it. I tried many different things to feel more alive. In each thing I tried, I thought I'd find myself, my happiness. At the end of the day, I was still praying my silent prayer with no response from God yet again. I felt unworthy, undervalued, and completely alone. I figured if I threw myself into being a good Godly homemaker, maybe I would be worthy. I wore the cute church clothes, made only healthy, clean meals, and homeschooled my children. I thought these things might bring me joy at some point. On the outside you'd think I was happy as could be, but I couldn't keep hiding my pain behind cute clothes and healthy homemade meals.

I began searching for truths, and little by little, I found pieces of myself. Like Humpty Dumpty, I put myself back together again. Humpty Dumpty did get put back together, right? For the sake of this story, let's say the king's men couldn't put him back together, so he put himself back together. I began putting myself back together with many truths I learned from wise friends, spiritual teachers, motivational speakers, and eventually, when I was ready, from the truths within. I began to hear messages that told me I was worthy; I had value; I hadn't been abandoned. These warmed my heart and gave me hope. I continued to search for more truths, yet I was a bit afraid that what I was hearing would take me down another disappointing road. How could I trust my thoughts and what felt true to me?

Predictive dreams and insight from intuitive thoughts started flowing through me. This is when I found the Divine. I am certain the Divine is God, but for me, it felt different. The Divine spoke to me, guided me, and supported me. The God I was taught judged me, abandoned me, and left me dying inside in complete silence. What was the difference? Was it because I started looking within instead of outside of myself? Maybe. All I knew was that I finally started to understand the needs of my soul—I felt revived—and that felt like something I could trust.

People thought I was crazy, and there were times I also wondered if I'd gone nuts. As I continued to go within and find Divine truths, I started setting boundaries and standing up for myself. I learned who I was and my worth. I used many methods to get to know myself better: astrology, retreats, healing sessions, music, and moments of sacred medicine helped me find pieces of my soul. Slowly, I began to feel alive again. I quit saying my silent prayer at night and started looking forward to being seen and heard. Like my version of Humpty Dumpty, I climbed back up the wall I fell from and started over again.

Looking back on my life now, I see the balance. I had to endure some difficult times to truly be ready to find my inner truths. Sometimes balance looks like chaos, but in the end, it brings purification and renewal. Some of my most painful memories motivated me to help others who have experienced similar hardships. I guess that's the balance of the pain. Before we can help others with their pain, we must first heal our own pain.

Becoming free from the limitations that are attached to our past helps us move forward in our Divinity. The patterns from my past haunted me and caused me to lose pieces of myself until I completely lost my identity. Like many others, I began to think I was the pain and felt all alone. Through my struggle, I learned I'm never alone. I have a support system. A Divine Consciousness that always guides me because it resides within me and within all of us! To ease my loneliness, I had to learn how to tap into my Divine Consciousness.

You can let go of the pain and limitations by working with the awareness that comes from the struggle. When the negative thoughts, false beliefs, and old emotions are cleared, you are left with the Divinity within. Many of us doubt ourselves and close off the deep inner truths because we feel judged, rejected, or weird. We must face these emotions to move forward and become our true self.

THE MEDICINE

"Finding your own sacred
Divinity will unlock ecstatic living in your everyday life."

If you feel lost or disconnected from your Divinity, then take one step at a time towards trusting yourself. I started with meditation. I once heard meditation means to become familiar with. If that is true, then by meditating we become familiar with ourselves and our own Divinity. I opened this chapter with one of my sacred practices of meditative writing. Meditation is about letting go of control and surrendering to your inner guidance. It has been proven to relieve stress and bring more peace and clarity to the mind. Remember, it's not about doing things a certain way; it's about the journey to your sacred truths. Your Divinity will guide you to your sacred medicine and help you do things your way.

Here's how I recommend practicing meditative writing. First, find a special journal that is only used for this type of writing. Then find a sacred space where you feel safe and comfortable—nature is great for this, but you can also find a quiet space in your home and set it up with candles, crystals, incense, or other soothing objects. Before you enter meditation, energetically cleanse your space and yourself to ensure the energy around you is cleared and ready to enter into sacred medicine. Allow yourself to tap in by connecting to your heart and then listen, feel, sense your soul, your Divinity, that place within that is free from the constraints of this world. Listen to your heart by quieting your mind. Once you feel fully connected, begin to write. Don't think about what you're writing; feel the writing. You'll be amazed at what flows through you. Just when you think you're finished writing, push through the resistance and allow your hand to continue to flow. This is typically when a powerful message or deep emotion emerges. Releasing these emotions stored in your energy field is crucial to connecting to more of your Divinity.

Inner balance comes when you connect to your whole being through some type of activity. It may be a celebration, a meditation, a meal— anything that has meaning to you. Sometimes this means taking time to feel the chaos, the shadow, and the emotions that need to be seen, processed, and released. It's all part of the balancing process.

EVERYDAY SACRED MEDICINE

Finding your own sacred Divinity will unlock ecstatic living in your everyday life. What is sacred to you? What warms your heart and causes it to flutter? It doesn't have to be something big. In fact, my definition of sacred is very simple:

Simple

Acts

Create

Real

Experiences for

Divinity

Sacred Medicine can easily be applied to your life. If you do simple acts to declare sacredness, then it is sacred. You may set aside a garment that you only wear for special occasions—that is a simple act declaring sacredness. You may have a special candle that you light during rituals—that is a sacred candle. These things make you feel special or connect you to more than just the physical. Sacredness connects you to your inner self. Think of an outfit that makes you feel like a million bucks. Is it really the outfit? If someone else put that outfit on, would they feel like a million bucks? Maybe, maybe not. Therefore it's not the outfit; it's how you feel in the outfit. It's about you, not what you're wearing. The same goes for things you use in your sacred practice.

ONCE IN A WHILE SACRED MEDICINE

I absolutely love the Once in a While Sacred Medicine because I can draw from it for years. These experiences tend to marinate in my soul and bring so much more flavor to life.

Conferences, travel, and holiday magic can bring intense medicine in a short period. I have found that if I try to keep myself in a box in these areas, I usually resent them. Once my family let go of the chains of "you have to do it this way," we began to feel free, more connected, and had deep, meaningful experiences. It is extremely freeing to do things in your own sacred way! Be your YOUnique self and enjoy your sacred medicine.

For more in-depth resource, visit our website www.mysticmeadowshealing.com and click on the resources tab. There is a mystical adventure waiting to unfold within you.

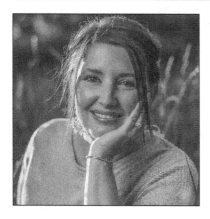

Amber's mission is to help others experience Divine alignment and find their TRUE happiness, so they feel supported and guided in all areas of their life. She believes everyone deserves to connect to the Divinity within by exploring their truths through sacred medicine.

Amber works with the blueprint of the soul to guide her clients on a journey of inner truth. In a sense, she helps you follow the map of your Divine truths to find the treasure within.

There is a bridge from your body to your spirit that must be found to connect to your whole being. Many people are lost on one side of the bridge, struggling to connect the two sides. She transformed her life as well as the life of her family with the techniques she teaches today. She is the co-founder of Mystic Meadows Healing, where she and her husband offer healing services.

https://www.mysticmeadowshealing.com/resources.

CHAPTER 18

FEEL YOUR WAY RICH

HOW TO ALIGN WITH THE FREQUENCY OF ABUNDANCE

Victoria Welsh, RN, BSN

MY STORY

It was two days before his 11th birthday. My son was in the kitchen ranting and raving to his friend about the cool birthday party he would have at the local trampoline park. "So, it's going to be you, me, Justin, Connor, Michael, and Alex," I heard him say. "You should invite the other Justin from Second Court and the twins from Fifth Court too," his friend chimed in. "Oh yeah, good idea. I think I will invite them. So anyway, after the trampoline park, we will all come back here to my house and have pizza and ice-cream cake and then everyone can spend the night. We can have a Nerf gun fight and suck helium out of all the balloons. It's going to be so cool, dude," my son said with so much excitement in his voice.

I sat just a few feet away, on the sofa, listening to their conversation. For the entirety of it, my stomach was in knots. Beads of sweat formed on my forehead. My heart was racing. My body was riddled with the effects of panic and anxiety.

From the first sentence he had spoken, all I could see were dollar signs in my head. I added up the cost as he added more kids to his invite list. With each kid he named, my stomach knotted up more. I knew the cost for the trampoline park was twenty-five dollars per kid for just two hours of jump time. His invite list was now up to nine boys. Stack on the balloons, pizza, and ice-cream cake, and it was all well over the amount of money I had in my bank account.

It was the middle of the month. I had about $200 in my account with no predictable income coming into my business. I had already burned through my 401K money in the previous six months, using it to support and feed us while I was building up my new coaching business. A friend of mine recently paid the rent for us. I owed several other people money. My credit cards were maxed out, and I was denied for all credit increases and additional credit cards.

"Breathe, just breathe," I kept repeating to myself.

My son walked into the living room toward me. He was reiterating his birthday plans. I acted as if I had not overheard his conversation. I allowed him to tell me with the same enthusiasm he shared with his buddy. I listened intently and gave him my undivided attention. All the while, I was quieting the voices in my head and battling the uneasiness in my body.

"What do you think, Mom?" he asked. "Does that sound like a good plan? I want to have the best birthday party ever since I haven't had a party since I was little."

He was right. He hadn't had a birthday party since his first birthday. I wanted a marvelous party for him just as much as he wanted one. I just didn't know how I was going to pull this off. My guilt and shame were consuming me. Fear was moving in and taking up residence in my body.

"It sounds like a perfect plan, buddy. I'm so excited for you. Whatever kind of celebration you want, I'm on board. I will make sure you have the best birthday party ever. You deserve the world, my boy," I assured him.

I didn't dare let him know that internally I was panicking. I would never have told him that there wasn't enough money in the bank to have the kind of party he was planning. I knew enough about money mindset to know that as a parent, I would significantly affect his relationship with money, in the future, by the way I handled money conversations with him in the now.

Besides, this was my money story, my money blueprint, my money shame that was coming up. It had nothing to do with him. He was just the child of a parent with a poor money mindset, which resulted in a reality of having no money.

My son walked his friend to the door to say good night; they were still talking about the best birthday party ever. I could feel the tears welling up in my eyes. I sat there, fighting them back, batting my eyes to keep the evidence of my failures safe inside of me. "Good night, Mom. I love you." He ran to me to give me a kiss and the biggest hug. "Thank you so much for letting me have a birthday party this year. I can't wait. It's going to be better than Justin's party; you just watch."

I wanted to jump out of my skin. My poor kid. He had no idea the situation I was in. I couldn't let him down. *How did I end up here again? How is this my reality?* I couldn't stop the thoughts.

The situation brought up so many money wounds. Six years prior to this incident, I was in the most awful situation with my money. My car was repossessed, my house was in foreclosure, I had filed for bankruptcy, and I had no money in the bank. It didn't matter how much money I earned during that time; I could never hold onto it. Money always found a way to leave me.

I thought I learned my lesson. It appeared my money story was still the same.

With tears stinging my eyes, I sat there wondering how I was going to make this happen. The last thing I wanted for my life was to disappoint my child because of my poor money mindset.

I had no idea of the 'how.' What I did know was that my money mindset did not belong to me. It was the blueprint I received from my parents, teachers, and the adults who impacted me while my subconscious mind was being formed and programmed (up until about the age of nine).

I spent the next couple of hours in my head, trying to figure out all the ways I could make some money in the next two days. I could not let my child down for his birthday. I just couldn't. It wasn't an option in my life.

I got to thinking: I could sell some of our belongings. I could ask a family member to borrow some money. I could create a new coaching offer to try and sell that. I was trying to come up with some ideas to bring in money in my business (new offers), but my mind was still wrapped around my lack of money, so I had a hard time focusing on making money. What a dichotomy I was caught in. The incessant thoughts in my mind were centered around scarcity and the guilt and shame I was feeling because of my money situation, causing me to stay stuck in my cycle of scarcity.

> *"We cannot solve our problems with the same thinking*
> *we used when we created them."*
>
> - Albert Einstein.

I needed to shift my thoughts and reframe my mind, but the more I looked at my situation, the more it reminded me of what I didn't have. I felt like I was stuck in a time loop. I couldn't focus on how I would make money because I couldn't get my mind off having no money. It was maddening.

The more I sat and tried to think my way out of my situation, the louder the thoughts of scarcity and lack became. It all came to a boiling point in which I found myself shouting out loud at God.

"Why? Why? Why me? Haven't I been through enough suffering in this lifetime?" My questions were to myself, the Universe, God, to anyone that would hear my cries in that moment. I dropped to my knees and hit the floor in utter emotional exhaustion. I could no longer hold back the flood gates. The tears were pouring out of me about all the years of struggle as a single mother and the loss I had suffered. My constant battle with money and never having enough culminated there on my kitchen floor.

Somehow, despite my lack of safety and security regarding my money situation, I felt safe in that moment to let it all go. I was on my knees, wailing, deep guttural cries, the cries of a woman at her wit's end, who just couldn't take another day, hour, or moment of her current situation. I continued on, screaming out loud, through my cries, seeking a response from someone, anyone: "Why me God? Why? Answer me! Just answer me! I don't understand! Why? How is this my life? Why does this keep happening to me?"

I think I was half expecting to hear God's voice and guidance, like the scene in *Eat, Pray, Love,* when Elizabeth is on the bathroom floor, and she hears a voice telling her to go back to bed. It would have been so comforting. It's exactly what I desired in that moment; to feel comforted, safe and secure, to be told that everything was going to turn out just fine. However, it became obvious after twenty minutes on that floor that no one was coming to rescue me. I was going to have to rescue myself. I was going to have to do the work to change my money mindset, and no one could do that but me.

I stood up from the kitchen floor, gathered myself, wiped my tears, and began walking toward my bookshelf. The evidence of my brokenness was there in a small puddle on the kitchen floor. I reached the bookshelf and pulled out every book that contained knowledge about abundance, money mindset, and wealth consciousness. There were four of them. I grabbed my pretty, red journal with the gold glitter pineapple and a crystal topped black ink pen. I was intent on putting myself in the vibes of abundance. I made a declaration that it was time to get real and face my poor money patterns and blocks once and for all. I was hungry to shift onto the frequency of abundance, that feeling of freedom and liberation from needing money, and into the overflow of an abundant life.

I spread the books around me on the bed. I don't believe I slept at all that first night of diving into this work. I was determined to uncover all my limiting beliefs about money and gain awareness around my thoughts. The more I read, the more I discovered that I was at the center of it all. I created my reality of constantly being broke.

The more I focused on my thoughts of being broke, the more I created my broke conditions. The more I focused on what I didn't have, the more I created a reality in which I would never have enough.

You see, it's our beliefs that create our personal reality. What you believe to be true in your subconscious mind is what will be created into reality and show up in the physical realm. As above, so below. As within, so without.

My feelings of worry and lack were so strong that this was the only place my consciousness was focused. Feelings and emotions carry a vibrational frequency to them, and it's our vibrational frequency that attracts everything into our reality. Your vibe (ration) literally attracts and creates the conditions and circumstances showing up in your life.

I knew I needed to stop focusing on my lack of money to find a solution. My son's birthday was just around the corner, and I still didn't have money for his party. I began paying very close attention to my thoughts. Each time a thought popped up about what I didn't have, I found a way to neutralize the thought. By just returning to neutrality, I began to have some clarity.

It was the day before my son's birthday party when a friend called to chat. I was so excited about the shifts I was already having that I shared my experience with her. When we hung up the phone, she electronically sent me $200 to go toward his party. Another friend showed up at my house that day with a $50 gift card. I couldn't believe this magic. The relief was overwhelming, followed by sheer joy, which then created a shift in my vibrational frequency. With this new shift in my frequency, I put out a new coaching offer in my business and two people purchased it. Money was starting to flow to me. I could barely contain my excitement.

My son had the most incredible birthday party that year. Four other boys ended up going to the trampoline park with him to celebrate with him. They all came back to the house for pizza and ice cream cake. It was the happiest I had witnessed my son in years and he never for a moment knew what I went through to pull it off. He just got to experience profound joy on that day.

THE MEDICINE

Abundance is a frequency that is always available to all of us. One must know abundance in consciousness before it shows up in your physical reality. We can feel our way rich by continually tapping into the frequency of abundance.

Just as lack and scarcity will continue to show up in your life by focusing on what you do not have, abundance will begin to show up in your life by focusing on what you do have. When you add emotion to that focus, such as feeling absolute appreciation and gratitude for what has already shown up in your life, you can speed up the rate at which that abundance shows up in your physical reality.

162 | SACRED MEDICINE

The key is to take your focus off what you do not have and place your focus of gratitude and appreciation on all the amazing and beautiful things currently in your life.

Abundance is in all things. It's the pervading frequency of all things. Abundance is in the air we breathe, the creative ideas we're inspired with, the number of drops in the ocean, the ever-present sun rays from the sun, and the vastness of nature. It's the sight that takes your breath away, the aroma of a decadent meal, and the butterflies in your stomach when you meet a soul-aligned partner. Abundance is omnipotent and omnipresent. It's the natural state of your soul, and it's your birthright to be abundant.

Three easy steps to tap into the frequency of abundance:

1. Start your day in profound gratitude for all that is present in your life. State a minimum of five things you are grateful for the second your feet hit the floor in the morning. This could be as simple as hot coffee, a warm bed, or a beautiful day. If you desire to shift your money story., then tap into appreciation for the money currently in your account (no matter if it's $1 or $1,000), for the bills already paid, and the creditors who trusted you with a line of credit.

2. It is not enough to just say what you are thankful for; you must feel the feeling of gratitude and appreciation in your body. This is the most important step because we attract things to us based on our vibrational frequency. All emotions carry a frequency, and gratitude carries a very high frequency. With the Law of Attraction, like attracts like; therefore, when you hold a frequency of gratitude in your being, you will attract to you more to be grateful for. So, take your time when you speak out loud about what you are grateful for. For each word of gratitude you speak, hold the feeling in your body of what it feels like to truly be thankful and full of appreciation for that person, place, or thing.

3. Look for evidence throughout your day of the abundance that is all around you. When someone lets you in front of them on the road, feel gratitude for the abundance of kind people in the world. When you take a walk in nature, give thanks for the abundance of trees and leaves and flowers ever-present. When you find a coin on the ground, be sure and celebrate the abundance always trying to make its way to you.

In every day, in every moment, we have a choice of what we will give our attention to. You are creating your reality with every thought and feeling. If you have created a reality you're not in love with, change your beliefs and thoughts, but even more importantly, change your feelings. Tap into the omnipotent, omnipresent frequency of abundance and feel your way rich.

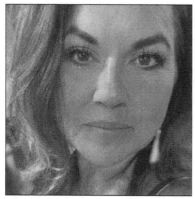

Victoria Welsh is a Spiritual Business Coach for Divine Feminine Leaders and Lightworkers. She helps women connect to their vision, message, and magic to build a business that is soul-aligned and prosperous.

She is the CEO of the Fierce Feminine brand and runs a group for Conscious Collaborations in the online space called the Fierce Feminine Leadership Lounge.

She's an energy worker, healer, and soul-code activator who is wildly obsessed with helping women activate their inner light and reconnect with the energy of the Divine Feminine to become highly successful in all areas of their life.

CHAPTER 19
LIGHT YOUR FIRE

ECSTATIC EMBODIMENT
TO FUEL YOUR DREAMS

Eirikah Delaunay, MFA, Somatic Sex+Magic Coach

"Let the soft animal of your body love what it loves."

– Mary Oliver

MY STORY

This is not the life I signed up for. I sat in traffic, craning my neck to see if I'd pass whatever the holdup was anytime soon. Sweat trickled along the edge of my hairline. The air conditioner in my car needed freon, and I didn't have the time or money to solve that problem today. I rolled the window down. My body was humming with stress as I did the math in my head: *Two kids—times $10/minute late for pick up—times how many minutes late will I be? Again? Goddammit.*

I tapped my fingers on the steering wheel, looked in the rearview, snaked my head out the window to look ahead, unable to sit still. I turned on the radio to distract myself. *Nope, not that song.* Flip. *Nope, not that.* Flip. *Definitely not news.* Flip. *I hate these prank call shows.* Flip. *Static? Why did it even bother to stop here?* Flip. *More nope.* I switched the radio off again, even more agitated.

I started running through the night's to-do list in my head. *Get the kids—Cook dinner. Finish the editing project I promised to have done yesterday. Bath time. Bedtime. Write the homework response due tomorrow and start the reading assignment for Friday's seminar. Grade at least half the papers my students turned in last week.* Traffic continued to inch forward, a brief coast in idle, then another stop. I put my head down on the steering wheel. *Okay, grade at least a couple of the papers my students turned in last week.*

Every day, the same stress, exhaustion, and short temper. Childcare pick-up poked every single button. I was always rushing to get there on time after teaching, especially on Tuesdays and Thursdays when my class ran all the way till 5:00. My husband's shift at the university café started at 2:00, so he was never available to help with this particular mad scramble, and he spent his late nights at the small independent hip hop recording studio we'd gone into debt to start, making music himself and collaborating with other local artists, so we rarely saw each other at all.

My thoughts shifted into a familiar litany of bitterness. *He's never available to help with any of the daily business of parenting, just like he's never available to spend time with me, not even sleeping time.* My eyes were stinging, and I couldn't tell if it was sweat or tears. *When we met, I was a sexy witch looking forward to a life of freedom and possibility, and now I'm just a fat, bitter house frau. Of course he doesn't want to spend time with me. *I* don't even want to spend time with me. There's got to be something wrong with me. Maybe I'm depressed. Maybe meds will help. I'll call someone tomorrow. This has to stop.*

The kids and I made it through another night on autopilot, eating corn dogs and tater tots while watching *Wheel of Fortune* to help them with their early reading skills by turning it into a game we called "The Alphabet Show" before baths and bedtime. I didn't have time for stories, but I sang them both their favorite lullabies, the same songs I sang to each of them when I rocked them to sleep as babies, and recited *Goodnight Moon* by heart to guide them into dreamtime.

I left the dishes piled up in the sink on top of the dishes from the day before, but I finally finished editing the book about the historical impacts of the cold weather in the summer of 1816 so I could drop off the heavy box of marked manuscript pages at the University Press the next day. *I deserve a break*, I told myself, so I started flipping through online chat rooms the same way I'd flipped through radio stations in the car, dipping into one anonymous conversation after another. I'd met my husband doing exactly this nine years earlier, and the lure of feeling sexy in connection with another adult—even faceless, pretend connection—was too much to resist. It was midnight before I knew it. I told myself I'd do my homework in the morning before class as I dragged myself to bed alone. The reading and grading I still hadn't started were added to the fog of guilt I carried, and I collapsed immediately into dreamless sleep.

The next day, between taking and teaching a class, I called the campus health service to get a counseling appointment with someone who could prescribe something to make me feel more like my old self. Hope buoyed inside as I scheduled an appointment for the very next day. Getting in to see someone quickly seemed like an obvious sign I was on the right track.

"What brings you in today?" the therapist asked as I settled into the chair in her office.

My irritation immediately skyrocketed. I'd squeezed this appointment in between a hundred other things, and I'd just filled out a stack of forms that included this very question. Twice. "I feel like I'm responding to my life inappropriately," I told her. "I'm snapping at my kids over nothing, and I can't seem to focus on getting things done. I'm constantly exhausted and overwhelmed. I'm either irritable or numb, so I'm constantly faking a good mood because I don't want to hurt the people around me if I can help it. Nobody wants to be around me like this, not my husband and not even me. I think I'm depressed, and I'm hoping meds can help."

"I see," she said. "That might be true, but I don't just prescribe meds right off the bat. First, let's meet once a week for the next month to talk about what's going on in your life and how you're feeling about it, and then we'll discuss whether meds might help."

At that point, I was willing to go through whatever process was required to feel clear, focused, and alive again. There was so much love and magic I wanted out of life, but I couldn't even imagine a path in that direction. I was in graduate school full time, teaching for the university, and working freelance for the University Press, raising two small children with no health insurance while supporting my husband's music production dreams. At the end of our month of sessions, my therapist circled back to my request for meds.

"We started working together because you thought you were responding inappropriately to your life and hoped I'd be able to prescribe something that would chemically help rebalance your mood and energy levels," she reminded me. "After listening to you tell me about everything you have going on these last four weeks, I have to tell you that you are NOT responding inappropriately. You are feeling exactly the way you should feel under the kinds of circumstances you're in. Your body's fight or flight response is being constantly triggered by the demands of family, school, work, and finances, and you're living in a stew of that stress without any relief. You don't need meds; you need to change your life."

"I don't see how I'm supposed to do that," I argued. "I can't quit school, or work, or give up my children, or ask my husband to abandon his dreams. And our financial challenges won't just disappear because I decide they will."

"I understand that it's hard to imagine a different way of living, but that's exactly what you need to do if you want to change the way you're feeling. Our bodies respond to stress this way for a reason—it's a signal we're in danger. It would be irresponsible of me to let you medicate that response away. It's telling you something you need to know."

I slumped in the chair, disappointed I was still stuck exactly where I was before. "So now what do I do? All the things on my plate will change eventually, but I can't just quit them now. How do I find the energy to make it through these challenges?"

"I hear you. Grad school and motherhood last a lot longer than running from a tiger. I don't have an easy answer for you, but I can point you toward some tools that might help you build endurance, like meditation."

Yet another thing on my to-do list, I thought.

"You have resources to draw on," she continued. "You're a witch and a storyteller. Where do you feel relaxed and energized? Use those images to reconnect with those feelings. If you feel like you can't change the outer circumstances of your life, change your inner circumstances. Visualize a different story. Practice paying attention to your heart and your body and give them pleasure when you can. They're not just a machine that carries your brain around. Listen to them."

Our time was up, so I stood to go, not meeting her eyes. "Thanks for your help," I said, even though I felt hopeless.

She stood to shake my hand and held it till I looked her in the eye. "What you're missing is desire," she said. "I've listened to you talk about all the obligations of your life for the last month, how hard you work to make sure other people's desires are met. But what about yours? Whether you can immediately make your own dreams a reality or not, the spark of desire can carry you through the challenges of getting there."

As I walked the three blocks back to campus parking thinking about what she'd said, my spirits lifted. There wasn't anything wrong with me. My life was hard right now, but it was the life I chose and would continue to choose. The sun was hot on my head and face, and a bead of sweat trickled along my hairline as I walked. I tasted salt as I licked my lips and had a sudden flashback of being at the beach as a teenager. I remembered how good the sun felt on my skin, getting hotter and hotter before plunging into the saltwater to cool off, feeling the gentle rocking of the waves, hearing the sounds of laughter and birds fighting over picnic scraps someone left behind. This was my place of relaxation and energy, where I connected to my body and my desire.

It was time to go pick up the kids, but I stayed with the vision as I drove. The air conditioner was still acting up, so I used that vision to shift my feelings about my current experience by focusing on my body's memory of blazing sun, heat, and salt. I let myself sink into the feelings of freedom and joy and sexiness at the beach—no deadlines, no obligations, just deep connection with the beauty and power of nature. I searched inside myself for desire and found a tiny flicker, almost forgotten. *What do I desire for myself?* I thought, looking for an answer, a path forward. *Can I give it a name?* My desire was quiet, but that flicker grew into a small but steady flame under my attention. The sound of children playing on the childcare playground through my open car window echoed the squeals and laughter on the beach, and I smiled as I hopped out of the car, on time for a change.

Later that night, after the kids were in bed, I stretched out in my own bed to go back to the beach as a conscious meditation, feeding the flame of my desire with the remembered pleasures of my body soaking in the elements of the natural world. As I tapped into those sensual memories, I touched myself slowly and tenderly, waking up my flesh from its long slumber, every nerve ending on fire, offering myself the gift of deep attention, a gift I almost forgot how to receive. Afterward, I slept deep and dreamed I was floating in water the same temperature as my body. I turned somersaults in the water, playing just because it felt good to play.

Big changes were coming into my life. This practice helped chart that course, and I continue to use it today. It is easy to lose sight of pleasure and desire as you hustle through the demands of everyday life, but sensual visualization is a powerful pathway to ecstatic embodiment as it strengthens the connections between your body and the natural world. It's a subtle form of spell-making, planting suggestions that help your body register everyday pleasures like sun and salt as pleasures to be savored, pleasures that matter, and fuel transformation and ease.

Tending the flame of your own desire in this way creates the energy and resources you need to dream big and achieve those dreams while staying true to yourself and present for those you love. The stories you tell yourself with connected attention and intention will create the fully-embodied, juicy life you desire.

THE MEDICINE

Settle yourself in a comfortable position.

With your hand on your breastbone, breathe deeply into your heart, feeling the glow of love that connects you to the world around you.

With your hand on your stomach, breathe deeply into your belly, feeling the heat of your own action and directed will.

With your hand on your sex, breathe deeply into your pelvic bowl, feeling the spark of your own desire.

This spark is the pilot light that fuels your creativity and passion, the flame that feeds your radiance and magnetic joy.

Take another breath, feeling that flame flicker and grow inside you.

Your unique spark of life force energy resides in your unique and precious body, and you can strengthen that spark, fan it into a roaring blaze by giving your body permission to fully embrace and enjoy the sensual pleasures of daily life.

Run your fingers through your hair, over your scalp, clearing all thoughts for just a few minutes, letting yourself be fully present in your body.

Gently caress your face, chin, and neck. You can feel tingles of electricity from your fingertips running from your head down into your arms and chest, creating a vibration of pleasure and ease.

Let your hands roam your body as you continue to breathe deeply, over your belly and sex, your arms and legs, rubbing your feet together. Touch yourself lightly as a feather, then more firmly, as your own pleasure dictates, as you relax and explore the beauties of the sacred vessel of your body, clearing the stagnant energy and opening the channels for the blazing powerhouse of your own desire.

As you touch yourself, pay attention to how your hands feel on your own skin and how your skin feels to your hands, enjoying both giving and receiving the pleasure you like best.

Breathe deeply into your pelvic bowl, stoking the fire of your desire to set your body alight with energy and power: power to connect, power to create, power to cultivate the life of your dreams.

As you continue breathing and touching, imagine yourself floating in a small boat. The sun is warm on your skin, a twin to the fire inside you. The water is crystal clear, and you can see the white sand through the sparkling water, just a few feet deep, perfect for a swim whenever you want.

Here, you are exactly the person you most want to be, with all the time in the world to do exactly as you please. You can hear the waves lapping at the boat and at the shore, seagulls crying in the distance. The air smells of salt and the warm fragrance of your own skin. Lick your lips and taste the salt of mingled sweat and sea. Alone in your boat, feel yourself rocking with the waves, your hands on your skin, pleasure, and power blazing inside you, ready to burst forth.

Know that you can let it explode into the dazzling brilliance of fireworks or hold it deep and hot as the hearth at the center of your Self whenever you want. This pleasure is yours, and it is always here for you, ready to fuel your dreams.

Slowly come back to your body, now relaxed but alive with the energy of your soul fire. Take one more deep breath, filling your pelvic bowl, and hold it as long as you can. Then slowly exhale and hold the empty breath as long as you can. As you inhale and return to steady, easy breathing, gently pat your body all over, anchoring yourself in the here and now.

This fire is always burning inside you, glowing coal waiting to be remembered and fed. Remember it in your daily life whenever you feel the sun on your skin or see it sparkling on the water, whenever you smell your skin, whenever you taste salt, whenever you hear the flow and lap of water. Perhaps you will be walking into work from the parking lot, changing clothes after working out, eating lunch with a friend, filling a child's bathtub. Wherever you are, whatever else you are doing, noticing the sun, the water, the salt, or your own body will reconnect you with your pleasure and power to live ecstatically.

Use this practice each night at bedtime to guide you into dreamtime. Notice the sensual bridges between daily life and this state of energetic flow as you move through your days, seamlessly feeding the flame of your desire and taking action to fulfill that desire while staying connected to your body and heart.

Let your soft animal body love what it loves and feel your power ignite.

**For an audio version and other resources, visit
https://desirealchemy.com/sacred-medicine.

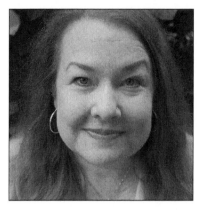

The founder of Desire Alchemy, **Eirikah Delaunay** is an initiated priestess and trauma-informed somatic sex+magic coach who shares her three decades of experience as a Witch and sexual rebel with others who are ready to unleash their unique desires and transmute those desires into connection and energy to fuel all their life's passions.

Eirikah's mission is to put the "fun" into "sexyfuntimes" by encouraging true authenticity, practical skills, devotion, and delight. She identifies as a queer, white, cisgender woman Switch who has enjoyed both long-term monogamous and polyamorous relationships. Both/and is her magic word.

A lifelong writer and academic with two amazing adult children, Eirikah discovered her spiritual path at 18, as she sought a tradition that held sacred the polarity of divine feminine and masculine, sexuality, and nature. She earned an MFA in Creative Writing and spent seven years as English and Gender Studies faculty followed by 11 years as a college vice president.

She has had the joy of more than a decade of connection, education, and service in the Seattle sex-positive community, where she has served as a "Tasting Top" for the local "Try It, You'll Like It" events, offering hors d'oeuvres-sized BDSM experiences for beginners, as well as serving as a guest educator/facilitator on topics ranging from D/s dynamics, sacred sexuality, and strategies for maintaining intimacy and connection in long-distance relationships. Her erotic writing has been published in the Seattle Erotic Arts Festival Literary Anthology for the last three consecutive years (2018-20).

She provides individual, partnered, and group coaching for people excited about using effective communication, magic, sexuality, kink, and/or power exchange relationships as vehicles for personal growth and bliss.

To learn more, visit her at https://desirealchemy.com or https://linktr.ee/eirikah.

Bonus resources available at https://desirealchemy.com/sacred-medicine.

CHAPTER 20

HARNESS YOUR HOME'S ENERGY TO CREATE A SACRED HAVEN

AMPLIFY CONNECTION, INTUITION, AND PEACE

Carolyn McGee, Decision Queen, Intuition Coach, and Teacher

MY STORY

When I returned a phone call on Easter Sunday, I had no idea how much my life would change. My friend and mentor Alan with his husband Jim typically called for holidays or just to say "hi." Alan usually called with Jim standing by, so when Jim left the message, "This is Jim, Alan's husband, the guy who reminds you of your dad," I knew something was wrong.

When I called back, Jim asked me if I was sitting down, my breath shortened, and my anxiety started to rise. His next words rocked my world, "Alan's dead." I immediately went into shock and disbelief. Then Jim asked me to help him notify other friends, and I went into doing mode versus feeling the immense loss.

The next few weeks were a blur between being consoled by friends and being the consoler. Alan helped me relearn how to be present to emotions, be the witness, and surrender so that the emotions flow through my body versus being trapped. I grieved deeply and was grateful for my ability to feel emotions and for the sanctity of my home and the sacred haven I created.

As I grieved for Alan, I found myself re-grieving the death of my father from almost ten years ago. When my dad died, I didn't know how to feel the emotion without becoming overwhelmed and paralyzed. I shut the emotion down, and it became embedded in my body instead of flowing through. Being present to and allowing the emotions of Alan's death gave me the gift of feeling the pain of my dad's death at a new level of awareness.

Four months prior, I followed my angel guidance/intuition and moved from Massachusetts to North Carolina. For most of my life, I joked about being a southern girl trapped in the north. At a very deep level, I knew that the energy of northern New York, where I grew up through college, and Massachusetts, where I lived over 30 years, was not supportive of who I am at a soul level.

Yet, it was a big leap of faith and trust in my divine guidance to buy a home 1000 miles away from my community, business, family, and friends. When I stepped into that faith, life flowed easily. I found a home in Asheville with a flat backyard where I could feel sacred medicine energy. Three massive trees anchored the backyard. Much of my work is centered on balancing the divine feminine and divine masculine energy through our hearts. One of those trees resonated with the energy of grandmother (divine feminine), another grandfather (divine masculine), and the third with sacred ceremony. I knew I was home.

When I arrived, I walked through each room to clear the old energy from past owners to allow my energy to thrive, and to create my sacred haven living space. I used sound, quantum energy, essential oils, crystals, prayers, plants, and intention to clear out the energy of past occupants. Then I brought in and anchored the energy I wanted to live in and make decisions from. Invoking the energy of the four Archangels, I set an angelic energy grid to allow in only the high vibration energy of love and light that

I wanted to surround myself with. Details of my practice are in the "My Medicine" section below.

I purposefully unpacked my belongings and consciously placed my furniture, pictures, etc., to optimize the energy of my new home. I was very intentional about what brought me joy and what didn't as I unpacked. I took the time to hold items in the energy of my new environment and decide if they brought me joy, and if so, where they would amplify joy and gratitude in my home.

A big part of my sacred living is communing with nature. I have been a crazy plant lady my entire life and have plants that are offshoots from both grandmothers' gardens. When I moved to North Carolina from Massachusetts, I uprooted these flowers to bring them with me to root in ancestral love in my new home. I had just gotten my gardens dug and heirloom flowers planted before Alan passed, and I channeled my grief into nurturing my plants in my new gardens and being healed by them in return.

Alan and Jim sent me a beautiful arrangement of flowers in a massive vase to celebrate my birthday and moving into my new home. As I created my outdoor space and gardens, I turned the vase into a water fountain. I am so grateful that I shared a photo of it with Alan before he died. A part of sacred haven living is to always follow your intuitive nudges to connect with a loved one.

About a month and a half after Alan died, I had the opportunity to practice this sacred living process again when I had to make the difficult choice to let my soulmate cat transition. He was sick for almost a year and held on to life just to be with me.

PD was one of my greatest teachers. He loved unconditionally, reminded me that I am a pet psychic and that being present is a gift. He had almost died in November before I moved but rallied to move to NC and spread his love and energy throughout my new home.

He followed me as I unpacked, explored every inch of the new home, and loved on me. I felt his energy wane and his spirit build. I knew that part of living in sacred haven energy is loving someone enough to let them go.

The loss of his physical presence compounded the loss of Alan. Yet, feeling PD's love and divine spark helped me to continue to grieve and allow the energy to flow. It became a beautiful cosmic dance of loss and love for Alan, PD, and my dad.

My healing continued as I nurtured my gardens and created intentional energy focal points in my yard. I hugged the grandmother tree to allow the divine mother to heal my heart. My swing became my inner child playground, the fountain the place where dreams come true, and my fire pit a dragon's clearing cave. Each area became a portal for sacred medicine and energy movement. I knew I was creating a map for healing bigger than just my backyard. This sacred haven living became a vibrational portal for healing and activating my coaching clients also.

I was ready to share my magic with others in person and had my first solstice workshop at my new home. It was a big clearing and resetting of energy for me, the attendees, and my home. The next day, I noticed a black oily smudge on the back of my left calf. There was no physical reason for it, so I intuitively knew that this was an opportunity for healing something I had buried in my energy field.

Our calves hold heart pain, and my angels brought to my mind the furnace blowback in my past home years ago. My home was covered in oily black soot, just like my leg. That event was the catalyst for me ending an unhealthy romantic relationship. It was painful, and I vowed never to be treated that way again and closed my heart.

Over the years, I did much healing on my heart and trusting myself in a relationship. Seeing the black smudge on my calf gave me the opportunity to clear away the last remnants of that block to having a healthy relationship. I used my sacred haven process to remove the old energy and bring in the energy that I want to live in.

I am so grateful I have the tools and knowledge to move energy, whether it be positive or energy that doesn't feel good, so that my physical, mental, moral, emotional, and spiritual bodies are energized and open to a joyful life. Creating a sacred haven environment and using the clearing and amplifying rituals below will help you live a more connected, intuitive, and peaceful life.

THE MEDICINE

The medicine of creating a Sacred Haven in your home or workspace is simple and straightforward. This is a sacred ritual with powerful results. I invite you to be intentional and reverent during this process.

1. Clear out any energy of who lived there before, the energy of the earth including animal spirit energy and energy from before there were buildings in the space.

2. Release any trapped energy or spirit energy that may have moved in from previous occupants or perhaps hitched a ride with your belongings as you made your way to your space.

3. Set up an intention grid of what you want your space to vibrate with. You may want to have your home or living space resonate with abundance or clarity or positive relationships or good boundaries, or a combination of energies.

Having a clear intention will support how you set up your sacred haven living space. Take note of how your home feels before you start the ritual. Are there areas that feel heavy or uncomfortable?

Sacred tools: To start the space clearing and energy realignment, I gather the following energetic tools:

a. A singing bowl or chimes or anything that makes a ringing vibrational sound.

b. A sage stick with a piece of clear crystal quartz and a sacred container to hold them in. I use a shell, but a dish or plate will work also.

c. A piece of palo santo wood.

d. A small piece of selenite and tourmaline for each corner of your home. I put them in the four corners of each floor of my home and the four corners of the yard. Find something that makes you smile to put the selenite and tourmaline in. It may be a pretty bag or a glass container. For the outside, you will want to put them in a plastic container or baggie to protect them from the elements.

e. A new white candle. I like jar candles.

f. A lighter.

g. High vibrational essential oils such as a rose, jasmine, or frankincense.

Clearing Energy: The first step is to go through your home and open at least one window in every room. Light your white candle in a safe place in the center of your home with the intention that it will anchor the clearing and resetting of energy as it burns.

Then starting at the lowest floor, whether it's the first floor or basement, pick a room and, using your intuition or guidance, call upon an Archangel such as Archangel Michael and ask to have any energy that is not of love and light removed from the room.

Ring your singing bowl or chime in the center of the room and then bring the burning sage to the four corners of the room to allow it to clear any stuck energy. Visualize the lower vibration energy moving from the room out the open window.

Make your way from room to room on the lowest level to the middle level and the top level (if you have more than one level), repeating the same process. Ask your intuition or guides if there is any energy to be released in furniture or objects. Then use the sound to wake up the energy in the room and sage to move the energy out of the room.

Anchor in New Energy: Again, starting on the lowest level, put the pieces of selenite and tourmaline in the four corners of the house on the floor with the intention and prayer of clearing what no longer serves you and amplifying blessings. The selenite magnifies intention, and tourmaline clears and grounds energy.

Burn the Palo Santo wood so the smoke goes into the four corners of each room of that floor to sanctify the positive energy of your intentions for peace, connection, joy, and abundance.

Put a drop of rose and frankincense essential oil in your hands and rub them together, then open them to release the vibration and scent into each room.

Do this for each room on each floor of your home.

Sanctify Your Yard: Once the home is completed, move outside to the yard. The Archangels are powerful energies that are infinite, so they can be everywhere at the same time. So, invoke their powerful energy to clear and protect your yard.

Starting in the north corner or what is closest to the northern corner, bury the pieces of selenite and tourmaline in the ground and call on Archangel Uriel. He is the Archangel of the earth, of the north, and of manifestation. Ask him to clear away anything on your property that is not of light and love. Ask for his assistance with any goals.

Then move to the eastern-ish corner and call upon Archangel Raphael. He is the angel of the east and the air. Ask him to clear away anything that is not of light and love and to bring in and amplify heart-centered healing as you bury the selenite and tourmaline. If there is a relationship that needs support, ask him for help.

In the southern-ish corner, call in Archangel Michael, the Archangel of fire, the south, protection, knowledge, and truth. As you bury the crystals, ask him to burn away any doubt, confusion, anxiety, and fear and amplify protection, knowledge, and clarity.

In the western-ish corner of your property, you will invoke Archangel Gabriel, the angel of the west, water, and communication. Ask her to remove any energy of flooding or drought from the property, ask her to balance emotions, and bring in and amplify serenity and peace.

Walk back to the northern corner to complete your energy grid. Spend a moment in gratitude for the angelic boundary you have created around your home. Feel the sanctity of your space surrounded by angelic love.

Intentionally releasing energy that no longer supports you and asking for new empowering energy will make your home even more inviting, nourishing, and comfortable.

Notice the difference in the energy after the clearing. Is your home more welcoming? Do you feel more positivity?

I would love to hear how you feel in your home after practicing this sacred medicine. I have a PDF on my website that you can print to make this ritual easier. You can download it and other gifts at https://carolynmcgee.com/resources/.

You may also email me at carolyn@carolynmcgee.com with any questions, comments, or observations.

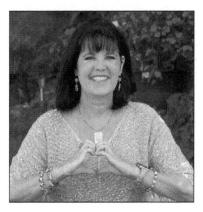

Creatrix **Carolyn McGee** is the architect of the Sacred Haven for Empowered & Intuitive Living Community which includes North Carolina retreats, virtual gatherings, powerful workshops, private coaching, and soul-nurturing VIP weekends. She serves women ready to connect with their inner wisdom, trust it to make empowered decisions, then take inspired action and discover the power of nature's cycles to create a life that lights them up. She has co-authored 10+ bestselling books, is a popular Radio & TV host, sought-after speaker, and blogger. www.CarolynMcGee.com

CHAPTER 21
FADING INTO HUMANITY

THE SACRED LIFE

Melissa Jolly Graves, LPN, ORDM, Seer, Priestess, Shaman,
Reiki Master, Reiki Teacher

MY STORY

This is it! This is that moment when all my spiritual work will be downloaded into the next matrix.

Creator, universal conductor, and my conscious spirit have been building, planning, copying, pasting, formulating algorithms, choosing my avatar, fine-tuning my frequencies, missions, and all I need to succeed as the character we created together. My spirit completed the tasks required in the spirit realm. The Creator approved my source coding design and gifted me a human body and life force to go with it.

It wasn't as easy. After designing my source coding, I had to find a set of procreators that matched my coding specification, uploads, and downloads necessary during my opportunity of life. They would be the frequency system that activates my light, lessons, and missions that lead me to my next journey as a human. Within them, they carry the right amount of happiness, love, and pain I need to experience to fulfill my destiny as my character.

Once I chose the right procreators, I had to align myself perfectly with the constellations, stars, planets, sun, solar system, colors, lights, shapes, chemicals, frequencies, and tone, so I wouldn't damage the energy I set into motion to enter Earth.

I'm a part of consciousness now. Although I'm programmed to experience human senses, I'm still spirit entering the womb. This is the place where I will build my physical body. My spirit energy starts to take human form. I'm like a hologram attached to my procreators. Anyone in the spirit world can see where I'm going next.

During the transition from spirit to human, I'm met by two energy systems and two sets of consciousness, each complete with spirits from the past, present, and future. These are the ones I would call my ancestors. They are the builders of the DNA before me. I must build with them if I want to proceed with calling these procreators "Mother" and "Father." The ancestors have accepted me as their future, and I have accepted them as my past. As I prepare my physical body for life, they share their stories, experiences, and warnings with me. They speak about the places, people, and objects they've encountered along the branches of life. They share memories by passing particles of light to me through the waters of the womb. I breathe these waters in, they pass through my mind and heart, and I accept them into my internal data. They have now updated me on the lands, people, and energy I'm about to encounter. I offer them particles of my essence as an exchange for their energy.

My mission becomes clearer. I jump ahead and set objects and energies into places I know I will encounter during my human form. These are the totems I have chosen to activate different chapters in my life: some good, some bad. We learn in the spiritual world that pain is beauty and sacred lessons that inspire spiritual growth and upgrade our human character.

I have chosen a name for myself. I will be called Melissa. Melissa was the nanny of the Gods. She later was turned into the honeybee to pollinate the world with beauty and lessons. That is the frequency of energy I wish to maintain and uphold on the Earth. I'm aware of the physical disabilities this name will cause; I accept it anyway.

Months go by in the physical realm, but time is irrelevant where I am. I am part of the forever energy that helps expand the Universe and consciousness. But the Aquarius portal I chose to enter is about to open. The energy I gain in this portal will also serve my human self.

Creator and I have decided I'm ready to play the human role now. I'm ready to heal what the past has created. I'm ready to expand and learn more so my spirit may upgrade when I'm done with my human form.

I'm ready to give love, light, happiness, hope, faith, and security to those humans who need it. I am Holy; I am pure; I am unaltered and made into the most perfect being. I am a Sacred one. My mission is to remind people who they are and the good light they carry inside.

This is going to be so easy! Everyone is so beautiful and full of pleasant light from up here. I can't wait. I must go now!

I say my goodbyes; I look at the cosmos and consciousness I'm connected to at that moment. I take it all in one last time. I observe the universe around me and jump through the portal of life. I land in the physical body I choose to inhabit. My spirit and body begin to exchange and balance the atomic structure and particles it has just received. Sacred geometry is established. This entanglement of the spirit and body activates the energy of the mind. I now have a core processing center and data for my spirit to live out this human life. My downloads are ready, and I'm ready for the world to see my spiritual doings and what my image of perfection is. I'm ready to integrate my energy into the Earth and in physical form with all the other holy souls who have entered the Earth.

It's time.

My spirit closes its eyes, and darkness surrounds me. I hear many sounds. The sounds are swirling all around me. I can feel it pull my energy into the circular shape, like going down the drain. All the water and particles act as magnets, bringing me closer and closer to this gravitational place of living. The sounds become rhythmic, low pitches and high pitches swirling around each other but holding a steady pulse.

The water around me leaves, and the walls cave in. I feel tight and condensed. My skin feels temperature for the first time. It's warm and inviting. There is little water left in the place of preparation, and my body takes in more oxygen than water. The force in my body changes, breathing changes. Pressure forms at the frontal lobe of my brain. My eyes open, I see a light at the end of the tunnel. This is where I need to go to gain a life.

This hurts so badly!

Wait, who said that? What is this voice inside my head? It's echoing my thoughts. This is scary.

I then realize the voice is my own.

But where are the other voices? Why can't I hear them? I am alone.

I hear another voice, a cry, outside this cave.

What is that sound? Where is it coming from? Who is that? Wait, I know that voice. That is the voice of the procreator I am to call Mother; that cry is my activation sound.

I go to the light. I can feel everything squishing together.

Yes, I can feel it! I can feel it! This is my next activation and sign I am becoming human! OUCH. Creator never told me it would be like this. Creator, I change my mind; I can't handle this pain! Can you hear me? Hello. This pain is excruciating. Let me back.

I look up; I'm closer to the light. I squeeze through the tiny hole created for my entrance. Immediately the doctor grabs me. This is the first time a human touches me. All the emotions of this human being fills my soul. He passes me to the nurses. With each passing of them, I feel their emotions; I feel their physical touch; I smell their essence; I hear their voices. *I am here; I am real; I am human! I am no longer just a conscious being. I am part of the entire whole now, and I feel what it means to suffer.*

I cannot comprehend the pain, energy, excitement, emotions, feelings, smells, and sounds. It's all so foreign to me. It's all so tangible, intense, loud, smelly, hard to the touch, and bright!

My entire body changes, tightens, my lungs swell with air, and all the air feels like it's ready to explode. My eyes fill with water—my mouth trembles. I scream and cry. Through my cry, I penetrate the universal energies with my frequencies and make my mark on the world. My frequencies are now a part of the particle sum. The universe pushes back with light force. My consciousness shatters into a million pieces, making room in my body for something else, but what? Particles of me fly all over the room and exchange energy with everything I see, smell, hear, taste, touch, and emotionally engage with. I watch as the independence I thought I was coming with, disappears and I become a part of the whole.

It doesn't feel glorious. It doesn't feel sacred. All my source coding is coming apart.

The doctor gives me to my mother. She holds me in her arms; she looks at me, she speaks, she pulls me closer to her. The pheromones of my new mother are inviting. She is warm and soft. My energy changes and calms. The sweet, creamy milk I am given shortly after fills my mouth and belly for the first time. I feel comforted. I don't know her face, I don't understand what she is saying, but I feel it. My energy softens; this is what it feels like to be loved by another human being; it's so palpable.

This is life; it's not so bad now. It's a bit comforting and all too real.

I fade to sleep. During that sleep, I ponder my existence, the reality of what just happened. It is at this moment I realize this is not the story of Melissa; this is the story of humanity, the story of us, and the way we interact with all things around us. It's about feeling the pain, comfort, hot, cold, warmth, tingles, touch, and emotions. It's about the smells, sights, sounds, movements, elements; it's about the whole. All of us and everyone we have or ever will come into contact with; I am them, and they are me. It has been that way since the beginning of humanity.

That first day of life was both painful and exciting. It set the course for the rest of my life for the difficulties, pains, and comforts I would receive throughout this journey. On day one, I was helpless. I learned trust, pain, emotions, nurturing, comfort, chaos, energy exchange, energy balance, and so much more.

I learned this place is a direct reflection of everything and everyone our Creator has ever permitted to be instilled into the source of all coding. All Creator loved, honored, approved, and thought to be perfect prior to coming here, was allowed in. Each of us with our own set of skills coming together to this land of the living. Earth is a compilation of the soul's art, beauty, energy, glory, nightmare, imaginations, and past experiences. This is where consciousness comes to life and becomes tangible. This place I now call home is all about the action and reaction of two sacred frequencies meeting and either accepting or rejecting the energy around it.

Earth is where you're allowed to see how things intertwine, connect, mimic each other, and interact together. Yet each energy field has a unique way of expressing the whole and how we live, feel, and observe.

Flash forward, I am 42 years old today. I have learned throughout my years in order to acknowledge anything or anyone with any of my senses, I must engage with the energy of that living or non-living object I come into contact with. Through quantum mechanics and teleportation, I must break my own energy pattern to allow for the energy of the alternating object to enter my aura field/universal torus so that I may comprehend its origin. That object must do the same. When this interaction happens, we break our personal patterns and waves, adapt to the patterns and rhythms of other waves, and therefore cause a new rhythm of energy called "particles." It does this by a delicate exchange and balance of the naturally occurring energy between two opposing energies units.

Did I confuse you yet? Let me try to explain this. I am a see-er. When I see objects exchanging energy, the giver and receiver always share codes in color, form, light pattern, and sounds. The giver and receiver must exchange these particles in order to acknowledge each other's perspective of the alternating energy. If the objects deny the energy of the opposing unit, it's chaotic energy, therefore, causing a glitch in the internal system. If the coding is accepted, it's sacred coding and sacred medicine we can use throughout our lives.

Example. If I am engaging from the perspective of a blue circle and the opposing object is a red square, then I and that other object must exchange the colors and/or shapes to acknowledge each other. So, we may come together creating a sacred shape such as a hexagon to balance the energy, or we may come together with a square overlapping a circle. We may also blend the colors together and make a purple so that we may communicate in the frequency of purple. Either way, the energy exchange affects both of us. Because of the interaction, we have both modified our internal data, and we walk away with the particles of the things we encounter. We keep those particles as gifts we get to take with us in spirit.

When I was asked to write about sacred medicine, I had a plan, a story, many actually. But the more I thought about it, the more I realized what I might call sacred you may think to be chaotic. So, what is the best way to explain sacred medicine to you?

Here's my take on it. Sacred medicine is the alternating current of energy that harmoniously flows between two energetic objects. Anytime a sacred constellation, energy point, shapes, symbols, universal frequencies, and different ideas come together to make something bigger, better, and more beautiful it was before the encounter; that is Sacred medicine. It's about serving the whole. What is best for all. Whether that is happiness or pain, sacred medicine strives to teach lessons, wisdom, mercy, grace, love, and healing to all energetic surroundings. It doesn't judge or decide what is right or wrong for someone else. It's about connecting with another soul and realizing you are responsible for all energies you encounter. It encourages us to put away any inhibitions about our own life experiences, emotions, and worries at the time and tap into new experiences, love, support, senses, and the corporeal reality of it all.

We are all sacred. We all came Holy, pure, complete, without flaw. It is the chaotic energy of the things we did not comprehend that make us something other than what we were programmed for. Anything and anyone can be Sacred; you just have to make the choice to take the good and leave the rest. It's also important to know that some things can be sacred or chaotic and change at any point during our journey.

To sum it up, the Sacred medicine we all came here to receive is life! Somewhere along the way, we got lost in other people's versions of what needed to happen. But it doesn't have to be a part of your reality.

My life is sacred and pure to this day; it's the integration with the chaos I chose to engage with that makes me anything less.

THE MEDICINE

The greatest medicine any one person can receive is to appreciate life. Love it, embrace it, feel it, live it. Explore everything, question everything. Connect to as many people as time allows. Talk, listen, love, touch, breathe, smile, laugh, cry, scream, move, stay still, be silent, whatever it is that you do in life, do it well. Do it responsibly. When something makes you feel warm, satisfied, loved, happy, overjoyed, gracious (all the good feelings), and it doesn't interrupt someone else's sacred energy, surround yourself with that.

It's sacred medicine in a sacred moment. Acknowledge the smells, colors, lights, sounds, shapes, people, items in the room, lock that moment into your soul, mind, and heart.

The thing about sacred things is they only last for so long before the magic is gone. Every light bulb eventually fades, but your memory doesn't have to. Lock it in your DNA, write it down, hang on to it if you can. When it is ready to move on, let it go and cherish it for the sacred medicine it was in your life. Cherish it for helping you through pain, tough times, loneliness, emotional times. It is a part of you forever. Your gifts in this life are tiny particles of the moments that made life worth living.

You are the sacred medicine. You are intertwined with all energetic matter. Be the thing you want others to feel, let go of the things that do not serve you, at any time your thoughts can change the algorithms of your human consciousness. Learn from the mistakes of others, thank them for doing what you don't have to.

Appreciate everything. You came here to experience; test what you like and don't like. If you don't like something, walk away. If it follows or comes back, take the lessons it offers; lessons are still sacred medicine.

You are love; you are a good light; you are pure and perfect. Nothing is bad; it is just chaotic. Every storm is beautiful and chaotic; learn from it, know the calm will come. Above all, remember the imperfect can be 'IMperfect' with a little change of energy.

Namaste.

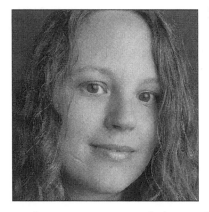

Melissa is the one-of-a-kind associative thinker who has the ability to visibly see and feel energy. In 1979 she was born a healer, but she didn't start her journey until 2006, when she became an LPN. She practiced several fields to include Behavioral Health, TCU, Alzheimer's, Mental Health, Senior Care, and Chemical Dependency. While working for Hazelden, she was called to do a different type of healing. Through meditation, prayer, and the guidance of her Angels and teachers, Melissa was taught how to do faith healing. She furthered her training in energy healing with schooling. In 2012 she started the study of Reiki. In 2015 she became a Reiki Master and Teacher. From there, she went on to train in the arts of Qigong, Kundalini, Shamanism, DNA healings, genetic modification, source coding, spiritual counseling, and quantum and frequency healing and has had the privilege to work with native healers. Currently, she holds 24 healing modalities.

In 2015 Melissa opened the doors to her business, Euphoric Source, which has received many awards. In 2016 Melissa was one of the 30 people in the United States asked to speak at the National Symposium for Holistic Arts Practitioners held at Harvard University. From 2016-2018 she hosted her own radio show called Euphoria Radio, where she began to learn how to communicate with people about her abilities. Soon after that Melissa was on Local Insider TV for being one of the most effective healers in the state of Minnesota. From 2017-2019 she was busy working in many temples, hosting ceremonies and spiritual events. Currently, Melissa is healing, teaching, advising, hosting spiritual events, writing her books, doing a documentary, running her business and science lab, being a mom and wife, and living life to the fullest. More information at https://www.euphoricsource.com/resources

CHAPTER 22

THE RITE OF THE WOMB

YOU ARE THE CREATOR
OF YOUR DESTINIES

Dr. Stephanie Rae Grenier, DC, FICPA

MY STORY
FROM POVERTY TO PROSPERITY MINDSET
FROM FEAR TO FREEDOM LIFESTYLE
FROM TRAGEDY TO TRIUMPH

I was a finicky eater and still am. Mom would not allow me to leave the table until my plate was clean, which felt like torture, as I wasn't fond of her cooking. My brother jested, "There are starving children in Biafra!" One night, after the table was cleared, I sat alone in despair, staring at my heaping bowl of hamburger casserole, retching from stewed tomatoes. My dad shockingly stood up to Mom, "Can't you see she's gagging?! Let her go!" *Hallelujah!* I swiftly escaped downstairs to my room. Nowadays, gratefully, I eat as much as I want of whatever I want.

My dad was my hero; there was always hope he'd come to my rescue, even when he couldn't. Except for one horrible summer, he was away getting his Masters. I seriously feared for my life because Dad wasn't there to save me. My mom's mom came to help take care of us six siblings ranging from about six to twelve years old. What a nightmare! I could never have imagined; *oh no! Mom's mean, just like her mom! I will NEVER be like them!*

It seemed I was always in trouble with my mom for something I didn't do. The punishment far outweighed the crime. I felt abused. I knew I was a good kid, smart, fun, funny, well-behaved, for the most part. I don't know why she couldn't see that! I figured she didn't like kids. It seemed like *she wasn't happy unless she was making everyone else miserable.* I stayed as far from her negative vibes as possible. I did, however, do my best to excel in life because I knew I could. I wanted to be proud of myself and please my dad.

Much like my relationship with my mother, my relationship with money was precarious at best. Despite being children of educators, like most people, we were not taught how money works.

As I reflect on where my old poverty mindset may have come from, despite the fact we weren't poor, and I didn't feel poor, my mother controlled the purse strings tightly. She was stingy and ornery, like Scrooge. When I wanted popcorn at my brothers' basketball games, I knew better than to ask Mom. Dad would cheerfully dig into his pocket, pull out a quarter and hand it to me with smiling eyes and a laugh! Rejoice! Popcorn! Simple pleasures indeed.

As a school superintendent, my dad had one week each summer for his annual fishing trip to Canada, an eternity to me. So elated upon his return, I couldn't wait for his bear hug as he rubbed his bristly facial growth on my tender cheeks, scraping them red and raw. Then, nearly drooling in anticipation as if he was slurping a juicy musk melon, he gave me some Canadian coins to add to my collection, which I proudly stored in a small Charles Chips tin. I sorted pennies to see what years I was missing and what was the oldest. I was careful to save wheat pennies and Canadian coins because they were unique and special to me.

In 1976, to commemorate the bicentennial, Dad proudly bought a booklet of two-dollar bills with an American flag cover. A couple of times, I'd sneak in his closet and peel off a crisp bill rubbing in my fingertips. *Surely, he wouldn't miss a couple.* But one day, I went back for another, and there was only one two-dollar bill left. The guilt and shame were overwhelming! *How did I become such a little klepto?* Apparently, I wasn't the only one, as Dad didn't intend to spend any.

A tidbit, I loved Boyer peanut butter cups and collected the cardboard coins inside to buy more. Blame it on a powerful sugar addiction.

Once I got into college, I was the skinniest I've been since from sheer poverty. I worked and played bluegrass to keep myself afloat. Senior year, my in-laws sent us five dollars a week, with which we bought a sack of potatoes and ate a baker for dinner every night. But a marriage to a cheater doesn't last long, so upon graduation and divorce, I moved to California with fifty dollars in my pocket and stayed with my sister's sweet young family temporarily.

Three years later, my fiancé and I moved to Massachusetts to help raise his girls and start our own family. I was seven months pregnant when I discovered chiropractic. We moved down to Atlanta for chiropractic school with nothing but admission papers, AJC job ads, our three-year-old boy, and fifty dollars. Yet another leap of faith.

While attending Life University, my work-study job was playing saxophone in the pep band for minimum wage. I meant to play guitar and sing in coffee houses, so be specific when you set your goals! Upon graduation three and a half years later, we bought our first house and settled into our new home and community. The police chief recruited me to run for mayor, despite my dad's frankness, "It's a thankless job."

The same month I was sworn in, I opened my new practice and learned to run both a business and a city simultaneously. That was a four-year battle I wouldn't wish on anyone. I thought I was handling difficult egos, rampant corruption, vicious smear campaigns, and lazy, lying staff rather well for a couple of years. I called Dad when the council wouldn't approve a much-needed planning retreat, "I don't see why they don't get it!" Paraphrasing him more PC, he meant *when you relate to people where they're at on their level; you'll learn to appeal to them better.* And I found surrounding myself with people who are smarter than me is a key to success.

Meanwhile, back at the office, I asked my chiropractic staff weekly how the billing was going. "Oh, it's coming along, we're figuring it out, we're getting there." I called them "my angels," so grateful and relieved they were handling my business. Once I realized they were *not* getting the billing done and I took it over, the insurance companies denied claims over a year old, and I lost over $300,000 my first year in practice. Obviously, I was not paying attention; I was devastated.

Once the four-year mayoral term was completed with the official Planning Report in place, in the thick of peri-menopausal emotional meltdown, I walked away from it all. I left the city, my practice, and my 15-year marriage to a wonderful man who had addiction problems I no longer had the capacity or desire to deal with because he didn't either. Understandably, my teenage son chose to stay in his home with his dad. And my dad died! I lost my three favorite men in one month. I was literally sick to my stomach. I felt broken. Broken-hearted. Helpless. Hopeless. Homeless.

I went to work with a successful chiropractor, a musician friend, whom I thought could teach me how to run a successful practice. It was a lesson in how to be taken advantage of. Three years later, when I left mid-negotiation because I didn't trust him to be fair, I took another harsh lesson on being taken advantage of for three more years with another chiropractor. And yet another, whose office manager set me up to fail. *Am I a slow learner? How do I stand up for myself?*

After floundering for a while, I finally opened another office. All it took was one vindictive disgruntled ex whose marriage proposal I declined, to sabotage everything in my life, including my practice, office, computer, network, residence, band, and he went after my license too! I lost everything except my license and son and was about to be on the street. Let me tell you emphatically, "Be careful who you let in your life! There are snakes out there." I used to be so trusting; now I am cautious. And I was finally forced to learn boundaries.

It's hard to see the good lesson when we're amidst disaster. However, the miracles that arise on the other side are priceless blessings when we focus on what's important. I ended up going into hiding on a friend's boat until I bought my own for next to nothing at an auction. There's nothing like being rocked to sleep and waking up on the water, seeing sunrise and sunset over the lake, simply gorgeous and serene. I became a mobile chiropractor and sang and played guitar using natural resonant healing frequencies as music therapy for hospice—instant soul gratification.

Mom and Dad made me, the DC, and my CPA brother their medical and financial power of attorneys. Our widowed mother remarried to a man who spent 25 years in prison for securities fraud. My brother and oldest sister were onto him, adamantly opposed the marriage, boycotted the wedding, and did not recognize him as our father-in-law. Five years later, after Mom's severe stroke, her 93-year-old husband got a temporary emergency guardianship which overrode our powers and ability to make decisions according to her wishes. He prevented us from moving them where she could get the care she needed near family and tried to take our family lake house of 44 years.

We spent $30,000 getting the emergency guardianship revoked. In the final hearing, the judge said, "It is evident your mother was an intelligent and savvy woman. She put everything in place to protect her estate from things like this happening. The prenup was signed, and her will clearly defines her intentions. Her own children are more than qualified power of attorneys. This temporary guardianship is unnecessary and hereby revoked." Sadly, within three months, my mom, her husband, and my 54-year-old ex all passed. Simultaneously, my brother discovered the transfer-on-death deed mom signed over to us, and our beloved lake house sold swiftly. I felt abandoned.

And now, despite my best early efforts not to, I have become my mother! Gratefully, the last ten years of her life, she displayed a spiritual kindness and joy after Dad called her out, "I think you like being miserable!" She exclaimed, "No, I don't!" And confided, "From that moment on, I decided to be happy." We forgave, repaired our relationship, and had intelligent, supportive conversations without judgment. One day she admitted, "You were always such a cheerful child, so easy." *Hmm, who knew?*

Since then, I've found countless ways to heal, attract, and embrace the vast amounts of abundance the universe has to offer, and pay attention, capitalize on, and appreciate the opportunities and blessings that perch on our doorstep. And I don't let the snakes in our house.

We must share our God-given gifts to enhance our world, our communities, our families, and our lives for generations. Ask daily, "How can I make a positive impact on every person that crosses my path?" Smile.

It all starts with mindset. Avoid stinkin' thinkin' that's doing harm. Attract abundance by sharing love and joy with others, and know you deserve it. Say, "I love you!" A LOT! And mean it!

Be grateful. Be purposeful. Success leaves clues. Trust the process. Take massive action because you create your destinies!

THE MEDICINE
THE RITE OF THE WOMB

There is a lineage of women who freed themselves from suffering through the jungle medicine. This lineage has given us the 13th Rite of the Munay-Ki: The Rite of the Womb. This feminine spirit of the Amazon jungle wants us to remember and share this simple and vital truth: "The womb is not a place to store fear and pain; the womb is to create and give birth to life."

This gift of healing and life belongs to all women in the world. Together we are the lineage that knows we did not come to suffer in this life but to be creators of our deepest longings and destinies.

Munay-Ki means the "energy of universal love." The 13th Rite of the Munay-Ki is so named to honor the 13 moons of a year, which are connected to the cycles of the womb.

RECEIVING THE RITE OF THE WOMB:

Once you receive The Rite of the Womb, you are responsible for sharing it with as many women as possible. You receive the Rite in person unless the Womb Keeper sharing the Rite is already capable of transmitting energy long distance.

It is vital for someone who has had a hysterectomy to energetically reconnect and reclaim their feminine wisdom and power. And if someone is pregnant, the Rite is a blessing that will gently inform both mother and baby of reverence for life and honor the intuition of the mother-to-be.

Men can participate in the ceremonies, and receive the Rite, if it intuitively feels sincere, right, and supportive to the Womb Keeper and receivers, as we all come from the womb, have feminine and masculine qualities, and are stewards of the earth.

SACRED SPACE:

It is important to find or create a welcoming atmosphere, inside or out, that feels inviting to you and the women receiving the 13th Rite, as that will also be inviting to the lineage.

Indoors: Create a simple altar that evokes sacredness and beauty. Set a nice cloth or tapestry on a flat surface such as a bench or table. In the middle, set a bowl of water, which is the most essential element because water will absorb prayers you'll offer to the earth for healing. To honor the 13 moons of the year and activate the alter with flames, add 13 candles around the bowl. Enhance the space and ceremony with flowers and petals on the alter, especially lavender and roses. Then use your intuition to check with the lineage about adding anything else. Ask a question and tune for an answer; remember that you are also in the lineage.

Outdoors: Find a place in nature where you feel the sacredness of life to perform the ceremony. Consider under a tree, in the woods, by a mountain, river, or rock. A lake is ideal, as it resembles the womb of Mother Earth, with whom we are sharing this healing.

THE 13th RITE CEREMONY:

1. You raise your hands and summon the lineage by saying, "The womb is not a place to store fear and pain; the womb is to create and give birth to life."

2. You activate the Rite within yourself by placing both hands over your womb and repeating, "The womb is not a place to store fear and pain; the womb is to create and give birth to life."

3. You transmit the wisdom from your womb to hers by placing one hand on each of your wombs and repeating, "The womb is not a place to store fear and pain; the womb is to create and give birth to life."

4. She affirms that she received the wisdom in her womb by placing both hands over her womb and repeating after you, "The womb is not a place to store fear and pain; the womb is to create and give birth to life."

5. Every time you share the Rite with women in your community, you strengthen its power within the womb. Let's heal our womb; let's heal our mother's, sister's, and daughter's wombs. And in this way, bring healing to our Mother Earth.

OFFERING:

It is key for every woman who receives the Rite to offer a healing prayer for Mother Earth. If inside, blow your prayers into the flower petals, place them in the bowl of water and release the water on the Earth, a river, or lake. If outside, blow prayers into petals or whatever your intuition guides you more appropriately and release directly to Mother Earth.

NURTURING THE RITE:

It is fundamental that, after receiving the 13th Rite, you nurture it for 13 moons of an entire year. To fully empower your womb, heal any imprints of pain and sorrow, and step into joy and compassion, start your year with your first ceremony using the following practices monthly:

1. If you still have your menses, then on your next cycle, you find an intimate space and time to give some of your menstrual blood to the earth. You can bleed directly on the earth, or you can collect some of your blood in a small container and pour it on the earth while repeating the following words:

> *"I release my fear so I may embrace freedom.*
> *I release my pain so I may embrace joy.*
> *I release my anger so I may embrace compassion.*
> *I release my sadness so I may embrace peace."*

Add any other words that ring true for you.

2. If you are in your years of plenitude (post-menopausal), then you'll do a ritual on the next dark moon and each thereafter. You create an intimate space to offer red wine to the earth while repeating the words:

"I release my fear so I may embrace freedom.
I release my pain so I may embrace joy.
I release my anger so I may embrace compassion.
I release my sadness so I may embrace peace."

Add any other words that ring true for you.

3. If a girl before menarche (first menstrual blood) receives the Rite and she wants to do a ritual, then she offers flowers to the full moon. This is because her womb is still blossoming and has not yet released her first flower. She can also repeat the words:

"I release my fear so I may embrace freedom.
I release my pain so I may embrace joy."

She is guided to say only the first two sentences so she does not become overwhelmed.

Then she is guided to say anything else that rings true for her.

4. Share the Rite of the Womb with the women of your community. Every time you transmit the Rite, you strengthen its power in your womb.

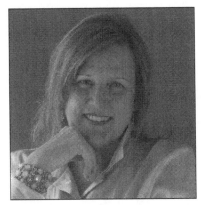

Dr. Stephanie Rae Grenier is a Mother, Grandmother, Chiropractor, Fellow of the International Chiropractic Pediatrics Association certified in Pediatrics, Pregnancy, and Websters In-Utero Constraint Technique, Author, Singer-Songwriter, Nurturing Artist, Sonic Healer, former Mayor, former long-term board member of the Georgia Music Industry Association, and an entrepreneur.

In the spirit of giving back, Doc Stephie Rae is on a mission to elevate, educate and empower communities with their right to informed choice. She uses her resources as Founder and CEO of Wellthness to create Wealth and Wellness Freedom Strategies for middle class families. And as Founder and President of Harmonious Heart Inc., a non-profit whose purpose is to share those wealth and wellness strategies and success principles with the under-served and our public servants.

Wellthness.com,

StephieRae.com,

TheRiteOfTheWomb.com

CHAPTER 23
EXPLORING SACRED PLACES
TO FIND THE SACRED WITHIN

James Kealiipiilani Kawainui, Native Hawaiian Healer,
Spiritual Counselor, Kahu

MY STORY

We make it a point to stay out of the way of the "rush arounders" (it's a word I just made up). I don't know what your personal experiences are around visiting sacred places, but mine are hit and miss. Most of the time, what I see, is a bunch of people racing to get there, grab a selfie *(Look at where I am!)* and blow through it all so they can be on to their next adventure. I see it a lot living in Sedona and when I was growing up in Hawaii. Their actions seem generally unconscious to me, with little reverence towards their surroundings, at least as far as I can see.

It is a reflection of our modern society. We have short attention spans and, for the most part, are self-absorbed. We consume news in sound bites, always looking for the next big thing. We've forgotten how to stop and experience the sacred.

As a Native Hawaiian Healer, it is second nature to me to feel the land and pause and reflect when I come upon a sacred place. I do my best to listen to the earth and hear the voices of the ancient ones who may have lived there. In that pause, I hear the song of the wind in the trees and the bird's gentle call. I notice the clouds skimming across the sky and the quiet murmur of a stream. These special moments become embedded in my memory.

While on a trip to New Mexico, my wife and I decided to visit Bandelier National Monument in Los Alamos for a day of hiking and adventure. I had never been there before or seen ancient Pueblo cliff dwellings and villages, even though we live in close proximity to a few such places near where we live in Sedona.

"Good thing you got here when you did. The park's already getting crowded," said the ranger at the gate. People, anticipating the hot day ahead, were rushing to get in. Even though it was barely 10 am, the parking lot was almost full. We found a place, parked, and got ready. We walked up to the ranger station, bought a site map, and started walking.

Walking over a short rise we were stunned into silence. *Look at all the people!* Everyone seemed to be congregated in a few of the main cliff dwellings at the front of the park. *This is insane!* They were swarming all over the place. It looked like an anthill that had just been run over by a lawnmower. *OMG!* We made a decision and went another way instead, heading further down the path, towards the back of the park.

The further away from the anthill of people we got, the quieter it became, literally and figuratively. The energy was completely different. It felt settled and not as frantic. Because it was a longer walk, fewer people chose to make the trek.

At the end of the trail we came upon a one hundred forty-foot vertical ascent to an old ceremonial meeting house and kiva tucked away in the cliffs above us. Always up for a challenge, we began climbing. One hundred forty feet may not sound like much, but when you climb a two-foot-wide ladder almost straight up at high altitude, it's hard not to feel a little daunted. *Just don't look down!*

As we climbed, I wondered how the ancestors had climbed these cliffs. I doubted they had ladders bolted to the rock that were OSHA-approved like the ones we were on.

There was no turning back. Several steep ladders and a series of narrow ledges were the only way up or down, with barely enough room for people to pass each other. We reached the top just as a group was leaving. We were basically alone, except for three others who were sitting quietly.

A deep silence washed over us. There was a palpable shift in the energy as we entered the cave. The sacredness seemed to be infused into the rock itself. No matter how many people may have climbed those ladders before us, once we were there, the outside world disappeared, and time evaporated.

In anticipation of our adventure, I had put my ceremonial kit into my backpack. It's a travel kit I take with me wherever we go, in case we happen to come upon a special place. In it are stones, crystals, and special objects, along with Hawaiian salt, tobacco, sage, palo santo, and cedar for offerings and ceremonies. We sat quietly in prayer, invoking the spirit of the land and the ancestors. I asked permission to be in this sacred space and in their presence, thanking them for the opportunity.

A peace settled over me and swept through the cave. A couple showed up and were instantly silenced by the energy as they approached the cave entrance. Very few, if any, words were spoken. I looked out over the forest below and saw the powerful beauty of the land around us. The junipers and ponderosas, like silent sentinels, stood watch. A crow called out, acknowledging our presence as it floated in the updraft. Shadows danced across the valley floor. Time stood still.

How many countless ceremonies and meetings have been held in this space? How did they come to find this spot? I sensed the ancestors sitting around us. Gratitude washed over me. I felt both honored and thankful to be in their presence.

In the distance, I heard the sound of a large group coming up the ladder. The moment passed, the energy interrupted. We knew it was time to go. As we stood up to leave, I saw acknowledgment in the eyes of the three people who were here with us. In that unspoken moment, we were kindred spirits, connected with each other and to this place. We would carry this experience with us as we stepped back into the world.

As we left, we passed a mom and dad with five young children in tow, as well as another group of people behind them. "Was it worth the climb?" the dad asked. I could only smile at him. There really are no words. *You'll find out for yourself and have the experience that you're ready to have,* I thought to myself.

This is the way of sacred places. We are drawn to them, sometimes for unknown reasons. And when we get there, we will each have our own unique experience. That experience is based on where we are inside of ourselves and our understanding of the energy we feel. What will the land or the ancestors be ready to share with us? Will we be able to hear what they have to say?

*****

What makes visiting sacred places so special?

Sacred places speak to a part of ourselves that is so deeply hidden inside that we may not be consciously aware of its internal presence. We sense the energy and are drawn to it. It awakens deep feelings. In those moments, we are connecting to something that is outside of our normal everyday existence. Spending time in sacred places is our bridge to God, the Divine, the Ancestors, Universal Presence, call It whatever you will. Sacred places help us remember that we are a part of something larger than our busy minds, the part of us so intent on unconsciously dictating our day-to-day habits and behaviors. Sacred places remind us we are not separate and that there can be Oneness with everything. They help us reconnect to this Oneness so we can feel that relationship, not only inside ourselves but in our lives as well.

I remember the first time I stood on the edge of the Grand Canyon. As I gazed down into the canyon and across to the other side, I felt the immense power of nature. It invoked a profound sense of humbleness. Hawaiians call this Ha`aha`a (humility). The land pulsed with energy. I felt the presence of the ancient ones and the respect and reverence they had for everything around them. I closed my eyes and felt myself soaring out over the cliffs with the crows. I heard the chanting of voices in ceremony, drums beating a steady rhythm in the background. The experience reminded me that the world was much larger than my insignificant thoughts and actions. At the same time, it called me to remember and appreciate the awe and splendor of our Earth Mother.

I've had many experiences in sacred places that have left deep and lasting impressions to this very day. When we are blessed to have such an opportunity, it can change our lives forever.

How do we go to a place and feel the Mana, the Divine Presence, and Life Force pulsing beneath the surface, beyond what our eyes see?

Here are some guidelines you may want to consider.

First, never assume it is okay to be in a sacred place simply because it's what *you* want to do! Always ask permission to be there. You may wonder, who am I asking permission from? You are asking the permission of the ancestors and the Spirit of the Land that inhabits the space. As you ask for permission, make an offering as a symbol of respect. Your offering can be salt, tobacco, cedar, or food. You get to decide what feels appropriate. Look at your offering as an energetic entry fee.

Once you've made your offering, listen and wait to receive your answer. Answers usually come in the form of a feeling or a sign from nature. Always be mindful that you are encroaching in a place where you may not be welcome. You are a guest; act accordingly. How would you feel if someone came in, trampled around uninvited in your home, then took something sacred of yours because they wanted it for themselves?

I've been told "no" many times before and always left without questioning. Learn to see the signs and heed the warnings. The ancestors, the spirit of the land, the animal spirits, don't take kindly to people who do not show respect. I've seen things happen many times in the past. People who got mysteriously hurt or ill because they did not respect where they were.

If permission is given, do what you are feeling drawn to do, always mindful that your ceremony is in resonance with the land and the ancestors.

Sacred places are there for everyone. Give others the ability to have their own experience without your imprint and energy. Out of respect for those that come after you, do your best to leave no trace.

THE MEDICINE

DO YOU SEE YOURSELF AND YOUR LIFE AS SACRED?

We toss around the word and use it in a variety of contexts, but do you know what it means? Ask yourself, "What does sacred mean to me?" Take a few moments and give this some thought. Write down a few words or ideas to help you gain clarity.

Sacred is not intellectual or mental; it is visceral. It's not conceptual; it's an energy and a feeling. To know the sacred is to have an awareness that something much greater than myself is present. I am being offered a glimpse and an opportunity to connect to its vastness, wisdom, and power. This experience is outside of my normal, everyday existence and connects me to the Divine. When I am in a sacred place or on sacred land, that connection to the Divine emanates from the very ground I am standing on and makes it easier for me to see and feel it inside of myself.

When I was standing on the rim of the Grand Canyon and in that cave at Bandelier, I felt an energy rise up from within me, sparking unconscious memories and a deep feeling of peace and knowing. This was not a thought; it was an energy I felt in my body. The sacredness of the land was now inside of me.

How can you know and experience the Divine in your daily life? Here are a few questions to contemplate:

Do you speak words of kindness, encouragement, compassion, and power to uplift yourself and others?

What you say to yourself about yourself matters. This bears repeating over and over again. Every time you use negative or disparaging words towards yourself, you are not seeing yourself as sacred or treating yourself with respect. *I am so stupid! That was a dumb thing to do. I'll never be happy. I'm just no good. Why does this always happen to me?* The energy of the words you use has long-lasting effects. They follow you and create the world around you to reflect your feelings.

Explore saying words like this to yourself:

**_I choose to be more aware of the words I use
and the impact they have on my life._**

Do you care for your health and well-being with loving attention?

How you take care of your physical form is another way of seeing yourself as sacred. You would never consciously desecrate a sacred site, yet you may be doing that to yourself every day by choosing not to care for your body. Proper food, the right diet, getting regular exercise, not constantly driving yourself to exhaustion are important factors that help support your well-being. *I know I shouldn't eat that, but I'm doing it anyway. I should make dinner and not get takeaway, but I'm too lazy to make the effort. I'm too tired to exercise. I'm too busy to go for a walk. I'll stop soon. I have one more thing to do before I can call it a day.*

Taking care of yourself is not only a sacred action; it is also an act of self-love. Here is an affirmation that may be helpful to say to yourself:

**I love myself so much and make positive choices
for my body and health on a daily basis.**

Do you treat yourself with reverence and respect?

Having prayer and ritual (such as meditation) in your life is very important. Ritual and ceremony have been used by humans for millennia. Prayer and ceremony have always been the vehicle to access sacred spaces and higher realms of consciousness, both collectively and personally. Quieting the mind daily is a way of connecting to our sacredness so we can bring it into our everyday awareness. Reflecting on kindness, compassion, love, or understanding helps us live and see what is sacred in our daily life.

If you haven't committed yourself to a consistent, daily routine, I strongly urge you to do so. I guarantee you will see results. It doesn't have to be complicated. Begin with something simple that works for you and build on it. You can start with just five minutes a day.

Here is a short meditation to help you get going:

jameskawainui043.lpages.co/self-love-time-out-meditation. You can lengthen the amount of time as you get comfortable with the process. Here is an affirmation that may be helpful:

Daily prayer and meditation helps me connect to my sacred place within

One of the ways you can support your meditation and inner connection is by having a place that is a focal point to hold your energy. Do you have a place for yourself that you've set aside, where you go to meditate and do your prayers? Having such a place helps create stability. As you keep returning daily to your sacred space, it will build energetically and support you on your journey.

Why do you imagine people are drawn to places like Stonehenge, Angkor Wat, Lourdes, or Giza, to name but a few, and the many other sacred sites that exist all over the world? These places are saturated with ritual and energy from countless ceremonies and of the people who have prayed there throughout the years. Your sacred space will do this for you.

You can use crystals, stones, or objects that feel sacred to you. I use a candle and light incense. I have a special cushion and chair. I will sometimes use soft, gentle music. You may have pictures of a teacher, deity, or loved one who inspires you. You decide what you want to put in your space; knowing how your sacred space feels will support you in taking time for yourself daily.

Two things are important here. One is consistency. The more you create this habit, the stronger it will become. It will become so embedded that when you miss it, you will notice it in the way your day goes. I guarantee you this will happen. "I notice how differently my day goes when I miss my Sacred Time." I've heard this so many times from my students and clients.

These are but a thimbleful of things you can do for yourself to create sacred space in your life. For more information on creating sacred space for yourself, reach out at: https://jameskawainui.com/get-back-on-track/. I can help you design a simple ritual that will support you on your spiritual path.

Creating sacred space for yourself is essential in these turbulent times. Every time you sit in your sacred space and give yourself time to connect to a presence greater than yourself, you will support and strengthen the sacred within you. The peace that comes will be beyond anything you could ever imagine. My love goes with you as you take that step on your journey to deeper awareness and understanding.

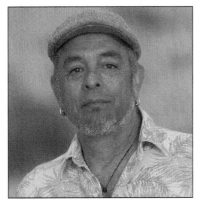

James Kawainui is a Native Hawaiian Healer with deep family roots in ancient Hawaii. Over Twenty years ago, James walked away from the "corporate world" and moved back to Hawaii. Since then, he has lived, studied, and worked with Traditional Hawaiian and New Zealand Maori Healers. James is the creator of a modern energy healing technique based on both ancient wisdom and modern medicine, designed to facilitate deep transformation. The effects are life-changing and help to reset the body to its Innate Natural Wisdom.

Results are often described as miraculous by his clients and often include:

- Permanent reduction and/or elimination of chronic or ongoing physical and emotional pain.

- Significant reduction of stress, emotional trauma, depression, and the effects of PTSD.

- Identification and clearing of generational and ancestral emotional and behavioral patterns.

- Restoration of *Your **Mana*** and the natural energetic flow of your body for optimum health and well-being.

- Re-establishing your Spiritual connection to ***Source Energy*** and Your Higher Self.

James works remotely with people from many cultures and countries.

He speaks to organizations, groups, and at conferences and seminars; teaching classes on Hawaiian Spirituality, mindfulness, meditation, and energy healing. James has a comprehensive mentoring program for practitioners and health care professionals that covers components of grounding, understanding of energetic boundaries, and development of an elevated spiritual practice.

James offers free 30-minute consultations: https://jameskawainui.com/get-back-on-track/

For information on Scheduling a Session, Speaking engagements, podcasts, or classes, Contact James:

Email: kahu457@gmail.com

Website: http://jameskawainui.com/

Follow James:

Facebook: https://www.facebook.com/jameskawainui/

Instagram: https://www.instagram.com/jameskawainui/

YouTube: https://m.youtube.com/channel/UCBLNjzVMSDhaWX3NxMPNTzA

CHAPTER 24
MIND BATH

SENSUAL RECONNECTION
AFTER MENOPAUSE

Lynn Olivari, CHT

"We are all faced with great opportunities brilliantly disguised as impossible situations. There's always a door, and that's how we evolve."

- Dr. Joe Dispenza

MY STORY

I've always been a seeker. So, when I had an uncontrollable urge to book a ticket to Cambodia, I knew I had to go. It was an inner longing. I was hoping adventure would inspire me. Channeling my inner Angelina Jolie in *Tomb Raider*, I thought I would find the secret under the ancient tree roots in the Ta Prohm Temple of Siam Reap.

When I got down to it, I realized I wanted to feel alive and sensual. There must be a mystical solution somewhere in the folds of my subconscious mind. That solution felt fleeting. I journeyed halfway around the world, expecting to find bliss. Instead, I was exhausted, depleted, and angry.

There I was, in the cradle of zen, hating myself. What was wrong with me? I looked into the eyes of one of my closest girlfriends, who agreed to accompany me, and wept.

"There is really something wrong with me," I sobbed. "No matter what I do, no matter how much I love my husband, my body feels NOTHING."

I mourned. I blamed myself. I felt like a fraud. The good time was over. I was done. Is this how menopause makes all women feel? My friend brought me back to the present moment and blurted out, "Lynn, look at where you are!"

I looked around. The late afternoon sunshine was shimmering through the carved teak panels. The patterns looked like symbols exposing messages in the light across the floors. The scent of the tropical hardwood reminded me of sandalwood and frankincense. It was earthy and mystical.

I looked out the floor-to-ceiling windows, with a view of the jungle pool just beyond. The pool's dark metallic tile reminded me of a magical scrying bowl. The water was dark and mysterious, like a reflection of my future.

The room had a huge clawfoot tub. Across that tub was a tray of apothecary oils and salts. A beautiful screen carved with Apsara dancers separated the tub from the rest of the suite. Despite the beauty around me, a festering feeling inside made me hate the sight of those dancers. The twisted female figures, bendy, contorted, the paragon of feminine beauty, elegance, and refinement, were right in front of me. Were they mocking me or inviting me to join them?

Frangipani and jasmine filled the air. It was breathtaking. I was surrounded by tranquil luxury as I sat there immersed in anger and desperation. I felt nothing but my inner poison.

"It's not fair," I blurted. I was bitter. Just past the menopause marker of age 50, I expected more from this phase of life than the disappointment that accompanied every erotic encounter I attempted.

The beauty of the suite just pissed me off more. I wished for younger times with my husband. We would have lost ourselves in each other. But now, here I am, on a quest for the satisfaction that slipped out of my life.

My friend looked at me and exclaimed, "Let it out. What are you feeling?" I sobbed until there weren't any tears left. When I finished, I was soothed by my friend's presence, the room's luxury, and a tray piled with succulently ripe mangoes. We nibbled the ripe fruits, sipped ginger tea, and looked deep into my mind and soul for answers.

"I want to feel alive again. I want my skin to tingle. I want that juicy deliciousness of the mango to be an everyday thing," I declared. "I want to have power in my step. I want my body to respond in the yummy-squirmy way inside I once felt whenever my husband looked me in the eye and gently kissed my mouth. Most of all, I want to truly love the woman I am now."

My friend confessed she also felt depleted and disconnected after menopause. I had no idea; she hid it so well behind her success. "So many women suffer in silence, with an aching heart in the middle of beautiful lives," she said. "My dear friend, we don't have to suffer." She went on, "Just because you've switched off, it doesn't mean you're broken. You're just switched off. All you have to do is turn that switch back on!" She lovingly reminded me that I already know how to do this.

"Girlfriend, it's what you're best at," she exclaimed. "Use your own hypnotic trance powers to zap yourself!" We laughed. It was a relief. She didn't miss a step, though, and worked to embolden me, "Zap yourself! C'mon, it's somewhere between 'physician heal thyself,' and the cobbler child has no shoes. Get your shoes on, Miss Lynn; you KNOW how to do this!"

I immediately knew I could. She reminded me of my work with hypnosis and how my clients transformed almost miraculously overnight. I help people change their reality all the time. I already know how to get to the root cause and change!

"If you were your own client," she said, "What would you do? How would you guide a woman like you?" It hit me like a wrecking ball. I had to stop the blame game and get over myself. I had to take responsibility and feel empathy for myself.

I asked myself, "What do I want to think?" Certainly, not the hateful litany of *you are getting what you deserve!* And, *you are not worthy!* Those thoughts plagued me day and night.

I made up my mind on what to do next.

I filled that clawfoot tub and selected my salts and fragrances. I slipped into the water and allowed my mind to drift into trance the same way I guide people into the mystical, magical realm of imagination.

I used my imagination to stir memories of sensation. It was like a daydream, but it felt real. Have you ever had that kind of dream where it feels real?

I was quickly lost in thought. I imagined the beauty of the Apsara dancers, the misting steam rising from the bath. I remembered the power that comes with dreaming. When we dream, we generate the same hormones as reality. We can use this to our advantage and/or disadvantage all the time.

When we imagine the worst, we create stress. When we imagine bliss, pleasure, and ecstasy, we produce the corresponding hormones. So we begin to start thinking about what we are thinking about. That is a process called 'metacognition.' Through trance and metacognition, we develop an advanced state of awareness.

My awareness switched on. In that bathtub, I identified the thoughts I wanted to banish. I shifted my thinking. It was magical. I've watched people find joy and relief from pain, both physical and emotional. I needed to do that for myself.

The biology of our bodies affects our emotions. We need our brains to make the right chemicals. Our thoughts drive that process. We can make hormones associated with worry and anger just as easily as we can make the ones for arousal. When we worry, arousal drifts farther away.

I started to dream of the pleasure. After all, this is an inside job.

I recognized the feelings I was having also were a problem for many women. Many of us start treating these problems medically at first and often don't feel satisfied with that as a complete answer. Our situations are different, but we want the same outcome: feeling better.

I delved into what could make me feel better. The one thing I could do today was to make myself feel better about myself.

In that bath, I reconnected to a love for my body. A love for being brave enough to ask, "Is this all there is? Isn't there more?" Then, I could move to the next step. I understood that the first step isn't going for the big 'O.' The first step is having hope and feeling good about your body.

I began searching for a way that could help women feel better. That was the key, feeling better. Better may not be 100%, but it is a step through the doorway of possibilities.

I found mysticism in the temples of Angkor Wat and relief in the sybaritic spas. I found answers in my bathtub. As I allowed my mind to drift, I found the magical mind-shift solution.

THE MEDICINE

The magic of this sacred medicine is that it gives your mind permission to ignite the pleasure centers of your body.

The thoughts we think shape our beliefs and our lives. It can be as simple as a gentle idea about loving the body you have so that your body can love you back.

The following trance ceremony originated from the learnings in Sexual Freedom Hypnosis ® practitioner training.

As we explored ways to create change, the first place to begin is with awareness and perception. All shifts really start here.

In the mind bath ceremony, I offer you a chance to ignite your imagination:

As you read the following passage, feel into it. Allow yourself to imagine the experience, then ask which of these scenarios you prefer.

You can choose one over the other. It's your choice which makes you feel just a little bit better. The structure of this writing is designed to entrance your mind. Later, you may decide to practice the ritual of actually taking the bath you create in your mind bath as a beautiful way to align mind and body.

Prefer to listen instead? You can download the full audio experience at www.lynnolivari.com/resource.

How to get ready:

- Create a quiet space free from distraction.
- Sit comfortably.
- Set the intention to receive this medicine of hope.
- Take a deep breath, soften your eyes and begin reading.
- This is a hypnotic script; allow yourself to relax and get that drifty dreamy feeling as you read.

Begin first in your mind. As you read, allow yourself to feel:

Imagine for a moment your body is a bathtub.

Envision yourself hopping into your body bathtub.

Getting into the water and methodically washing your body from top to toe.

You follow your usual pattern, you do it quickly to save time, and with little thought, perhaps you're even thinking about all the things you will do after your bath.

You pay little attention to how your skin feels, how you feel inside, the temperature of the water, and you don't really notice the smell of the soap you are using.

You do this the same old way you've always taken a bath. This is your routine, the routine you might be ready to leave behind, and the feelings about yourself you might be ready to leave behind. They may have served you for a while, but like this bath, that time has passed.

Then, when you have completed your bathing routine, you pull the plug and hop out. Imagine all that draining away.

As you dry your body, you feel refreshed and clean, but your bath was nothing memorable, and you probably won't be thinking about when your next bath will be.

Now, allow yourself to breathe more deeply.

Breathe fully into your body.

Feel your belly and chest rise and fall.

Breathe fully into your being.

Imagine for a moment that your body is a glorious, sensual vessel that is there to be filled with pleasure until it's overflowing with delicious sensations and feelings.

Imagine that everything you think,

and everything you do,

has the potential to add wonderful erotic oils and bubbles to your erotic bathtub.

You might think about your bath in advance,

luxuriating in the thought of how wonderful it will be,

how you might feel,

how relaxing yet energizing it will be,

will you be alone, or will you invite someone to share your bath?

Will you play music or perhaps just enjoy the quiet?

You draw your bath, noticing the steam rising as the bath fills the noise the water makes as it gushes into the tub.

You take your time,

choosing and adding in the oils and bubbles.

The special elements that will create just the right experience for you.

Perhaps you light candles,

turn out the lights,

or throw open the window to let the sun or moonlight illuminate the room.

Then you climb into your bathtub,

and you observe and notice how your body feels,

how the water makes it feel,

the sensations on your skin,

the scents filling your nostrils,

the light of the room reflecting off the water, the bubbles slowly popping.

You surrender to the feelings,

and as you do, those feelings steadily increase.

Breathing them in,

feeling them increase.

Everything you see, hear, smell, taste, and touch are like adding bath bombs of pleasure that fizz through the water, tantalizing you, adding to the build-up of sensation.

You wash your body,

the softness of a sponge or the bar of soap sliding,

feeling good on your skin, perhaps you notice the contrast of sensations if you switch to a brush or loofah.

If you notice a particularly pleasurable sensation,

you spend a little more time doing it,

letting your feelings and sensations guide you where to go next.

Imagine that you give yourself permission to simply wallow and luxuriate in your erotic bathtub, allowing every one of your senses to become intoxicated with the experience.

You can feel the sensations surging through you,

your skin tingling.

You don't have to do anything except enjoy it.

You're not even considering pulling the plug,

it feels so good to be just right there in it.

You know what happens when you will eventually pull the plug,

the thought of it is delicious, the anticipation building,

Now imagine that your erotic bathtub is so full that it is splashing over the sides,

the sensual pleasure is oozing out of you,

It's all-consuming,

you simply cannot fill it anymore,

you want, need, and cannot wait a moment longer to pull the plug.

You pull the plug, and every sensation begins to gush.

As it does, the bathtub is still being filled with sensations,

but as it flows through the plug, it is amazingly intense.

It's building into an unstoppable feeling that spreads through the whole bathtub,

your whole body filled and immersed in an intense orgasmic feeling.

It's a magnificent feeling, isn't it?

Your body calms, and the plug is closed once again,

your body buzzing and your mind calm.

The bathtub starts filling, and a residue of that experience is left behind,

slowly it starts to fill again, ready for the next time,

perhaps with different oils and bubbles.

You get out of the bathtub,

slowly drying your body with the softest warm towel,

you feel so alive and happy, looking forward to the next time,

perhaps wondering what combination of oils and bubbles and anything else you might add.

Now ask yourself, out of those two baths, which one do you want?

Which one made you feel the most?

Which one made you feel alive and invigorated?

I choose the second one; I'm betting you would too.

You are the only one who can give yourself permission for pleasure. It can start simply and grow in beautiful ways.

If you take anything away from this, it's a celebration of the permission YOU are ready to embody.

Moving through the day in every way.

Your feeling of pleasure grows.

So as you take this in, allow your mind and body to feel the hope that I hold for you in this writing. If your imagination switches on, if you feel the thoughts stir feelings in your body, that indicates that this type of work can begin to help you feel better.

If you feel anything at all, it's a sign that this could work for you. If it speaks to you and allows you a bit of hope. Then I encourage you to find out more.

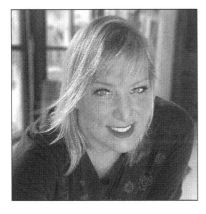

Lynn Olivari, CHT is a Mind-Body Connection Expert whose superpower is an intuitive view - it's as if she can see right into someone and know what is holding them back. And the good news is she also sees simple solutions to remove those barriers.

She is a Master Hypnotist and hypnotherapist specializing in Rapid Transformation. She studied at the University of Iowa and postgraduate studies at Aurora University.

As a nationally acclaimed presenter and educator, she teaches worldwide. Her topics range broadly from helping women connect to their sensuality to assisting organizations to improve their business through inside-out change.

During her travels, Lynn has visited local markets and taken cooking classes in 37 countries. She loves knowing 'the feel' of a place by experiencing the local cuisine and the vibration of the place by meditating there. She's a meditation junky and is proud to have experiences serving as a volunteer with Dr. Joe Dispenza's Advanced Retreats.

SIGNATURE PROGRAMS

The golden thread in Lynn's signature programs is that she makes things work better.

RTT Rapid Transformation Hypnotherapy

Gets to the cause, root, and reason for a limiting belief, then extracts it from the subconscious; and replaces it with the new empowering belief, thus, changing the results of your life.

This works beautifully for things like: Not good enough, not worthy, anxiety, depression, relationships, confidence.

Unlock Your Body Transformation Code

This group program makes any diet or exercise program work better. We get to the root cause to help you stop fighting yourself and find the easy path to better.

Sexual Freedom Hypnosis ®

For couples or individuals who want a consenting, confident, satisfying sex life in the absence of sexual dysfunction, guilt and shame. Rather than trying to get people to "logic" their way out of sexual dysfunction, hypnosis can facilitate lasting changes at a subconscious level. Hypnosis can be used to treat the many causes of psycho-sexual issues. Where the mind goes, the body follows. Hypnosis can help you do this in a positive way, overcome past trauma, change unhelpful beliefs, and make friends with your body and sexuality.

"All day long, your mind whispers
the words that become your reality.
Love what you're telling yourself
to create magic in your life!"

- Lynn Olivari

CHAPTER 25

YOUR LIFE IS YOUR MEDICINE

SIMPLE STRATEGIES FOR A LIMITLESS FUTURE

Darlene de la Plata

MY STORY

Once upon a time, I was a little girl who dreamed of being of service to humanity. Outwardly quiet and shy, I kept my big dreams to myself because although it was unspoken, dreams were very dangerous things that rocked the boat and made people uncomfortable. Being an only child until I was nearly eleven, I entertained myself by making forts with sheets and umbrellas under the dining room table and filled them with stuffed animals and secret dreams.

Life with teenaged parents was filled with the Beatles and picnics at the park on the 4th of July. They hustled to make ends meet, and I quickly learned to be independent. Barbies, books, drawing, and I Dream of Jeannie were my afternoon companions as both of my parents worked regular jobs and went to school. Being a latch key kid was a badge of responsibility, and I wore it feeling all grown up. It was all I knew, and it felt normal.

Watching the adults in my life struggle with their finances and emotions was a template for my future. However, I did not yet know these hidden secrets about my life. Children feel discontent in the unspoken. It translates into people-pleasing and walking on eggshells, so I became a bonafide pro. Keeping the peace was the name of the game as I watched the relationships around me unravel one painful thread at a time. By the time I was a freshman in high school, my parents were divorcing, and life as I knew it took on the disguise of freedom.

I left home at seventeen with a back seat packed with my stereo, favorite albums, and a suitcase full of clothes. The wild blue yonder of UCLA felt like it was a world away, but in reality, it was only 45 minutes up the 405 freeway. With big plans and a student loan, my dreams and I moved into the dorms off Sunset Boulevard with pre-med aspirations in tow. It was there I began adulting without a map or a plan, simultaneously exploring Greek life on campus and the Sunset Strip.

Life does not wait for you to get it together. It is more like on-the-job training if you do not have a worthy mentor. As a teenage girl on your own, there are plenty of volunteers to tell you how to live your life and willing to offer you their services. Like sharks drawn to the scent of blood, the opportunists smell your naïveté and circle for the proper time to pounce. They seem to smell the insecurities and fears we have packed neatly in our invisible backpacks, the ones we drag everywhere we go.

For me, that little backpack from my youth became a matching set of designer luggage I was reluctant to part with for any reason. While it was full of terrifying memories, personal defeats, justifications, and judgments about myself and others, I held onto it with a death grip. It was the devil I knew versus the devil I didn't know, and I dragged that mess around to every relationship and opportunity that came across my path until it became my judge, jury, and executioner. Over the years, my subconscious mind dipped into the suitcases regularly to fish out the exact limiting belief needed to talk me out of any liberating thoughts disguised as lofty, scary, exciting dreams. These contraband aspirations were flagged as risky, so I would move on and feel safe for a while until the urge for something more dared to rear its head.

Between working full time and dealing with health challenges, I found myself saying goodbye to college life. Through a chance encounter while trying to heal, I was introduced to the world of vibration, energy, and the unknown. Dabbling in herbal remedies and folk medicine had not prepared me for the rabbit hole where I was about to dive headfirst. During my very first session, I experienced remarkable supernatural healing, which opened my eyes to the mysteries of God's infinite power and the secrets of the universe. I am living proof you can be completely clueless and experience a miracle. At that moment, my medical mindedness took a flying leap right out the window. I discarded the world of medical doctors for the mysterious frontier of herbalists, midwives, shamens, kahunas, gypsies, healing ministers, and energy medicine.

After UCLA, two marriages, countless jobs, and four children, I looked around one day and had no idea how I had ended up in such a wild predicament. I was drowning and needed to let go of my matching bags for good or stay on the brink of survival mode, which was exhausting. It was the middle of winter in Georgia, and we were homeless. This was not the life I ordered, and I wanted to click my heels together to be anywhere else. Instead, I found myself huddled on the floor in sleeping bags with my children and my mother in front of a fireplace that thankfully still had the gas turned on. You see, we had been ousted from our home during foreclosure and had nowhere else to go. So we kicked out the AC unit in a ground floor window and crawled in like criminals to the place which had been our home for years. It felt like one more scene in a series of crazy nightmares, and for some reason, I was not waking up.

During my double life as student, mom, and employee by day, homeless criminal by night, I prayed for guidance and answers to reveal the source of my problems, which kept reappearing as failed marriages, financial ruin, abusive people, and overall struggle. I was so sure the problem was "out there" somewhere, and the more I looked "out there," the more confused I became. A pattern began to reveal itself, and as it turned out, I did not need a secret decoder ring to decipher it. I just needed a book store.

As a single homeschooling mom, I found my refuge in the local Borders. What was not to love? They sold frozen chai and afforded me time steeped in imaginings while my children entertained themselves with books across the aisle. The store hosted midnight Harry Potter book launch parties complete with hoopla and pajamas, and it felt like a safe yet magical place. I am grateful for the memories created there before it became a casualty of the online shopping era.

Books became my obsession as I uncovered concepts like consciousness, quantum theories, mindset, and prosperity. Doing a deep dive into the thoughts, books, seminars, and lives of people who had done it already became a priority no matter how far away it felt for me at the time. Discovering things like limitless possibilities and mind mapping felt like finding the Hope diamond. I gladly treated them like incredible new tools for my banged-up toolbox, which previously held herbal wisdom and street smarts. This was all timeless information but brand new for me, and it felt like I was on the verge of something great.

When I shared this newfound excitement with people who knew me, I could feel the eye roll before it happened. They were very quick to point out how crazy it sounded, along with all the reasons why it was not possible. After all, there was my lack of current resources, which to them meant a lack of future resources. And lest I forget my shortcomings, they had a list to bring me back to my senses. I was unceremoniously whacked at the knees, Tonya Harding style, at every turn, so I decided to attract a new set of friends.

Our greatest trials reveal our greatest strengths and gifts. When I look back, it is easy to see how my life was chaotic by choice because I did not have a plan. Until I did. For years, flying by the seat of my pants was my Olympic sport, and I had plenty of gold medals to show for it. One day that was no longer good enough for me, and I decided to start living my life with a map, compass, and an actual destination. I was crossing over into foreign territory, but there was something inside of me that was more scared of staying where I was, locked into scarcity.

Something beautiful was waiting on the other side of fear, and I knew I had to begin my expedition into the unknown world of creating my reality. I did not know anyone operating in this way, so I had to be my own Lewis and Clark and Sacagawea all rolled into one. The books said it was possible, but I must admit I wasn't sure if they were all full of crap, spinning tales to sell some books to the gullible. While all this crossed my mind, I had nothing to lose and nowhere to go but up, so I decided to give it a whirl.

The mindset of lack and scarcity is an underlying assumption in our society unless someone has consciously made an effort to undo the brainwashing that comes with an upbringing steeped in regular life. We are taught money is the root of all evil, we can't have it all, rich people are greedy, there is not enough to go around, and dozens of other pointless untruths about money, so poverty becomes our superpower. We are kept in awe of money instead of being taught how it works practically and energetically. We are coupon queens who start blogs on being frugal and how to make five meals out of one chicken. We hoard useless belongings because "we might need it one day" instead of keeping the flow of abundance moving in our life by giving things away. There are so many transformative principles left out of our early education system one has to wonder if it is by design, although that may be a topic for another book.

Life is precious and finite, and there are no do-overs. I look at how my life transformed once I decided to climb out of my pit of quicksand, and I am amazed by the fact it all started with a decision. The actions themselves were simple, but it was the mindset that needed constant tuning like an old piano. Since then, I have learned to manifest an incredible life with less effort than it took to live in fear, poverty, and uncertainty. This shift did not take diplomas or certificates; the change happened at the speed of thought. We are the ones who slow it down by thinking of all the ways it's not possible instead of just allowing an abundant reality to reveal itself. The truth is each one of us can change and heal our lives for the better, and it is never too late to get started.

For my life to change, I had to stop thinking and behaving like a poor person and a victim and start feeling prosperous and safe on the inside no matter what my circumstances shouted in the mirror. First, it became a daily practice, and one day it became automatic. I was relentless and took ideas from everywhere, developing games and reminders to call me out when I slipped back into lack. It made a lasting impact, and I could not help but wonder why everyone did not see how simple it was to change.

Personal reflection allows you to examine the good, the bad, and the ugly about yourself. You can stop there and do nothing, or you can move forward with a new plan. Our waking hours are spent explaining, complaining, or worrying about what we lack. Whether it's money, friends, time, health, freedom, or material things, moaning and groaning keep us focused on what's missing. These low vibrating thoughts attract more of what we do not want and create a cycle of defeat.

To the unsuspecting onlooker, I seemed out of my mind. When friends would ask me where I was going to get the money for something, my standard reply was "wherever it is right now," and I believed every word I said. Our planet is a prosperous place with more than enough to go around, so I would imagine some of it getting detoured in my direction, and it did. I changed my thoughts, and I became very particular about my words, guarding each one that came out of my mouth, knowing it would run off to create whatever I spoke into existence.

This carried over into every area until no regular thing in my life was safe from the power of my transformative words. I manifested a thriving health food store out of thin air, a husband from across the country, homes, cars, and opportunities galore. My vibrational medicine practice expanded to include visionary coaching and prosperity consciousness, where rock stars and sports legends became clients. I traveled to the Amazon jungle for an incredible journey that forever altered my existence. I owe it all to the power inside the seed of making that initial decision to discover something more.

Creating a life I love has been a remarkable journey and is so much better than the alternative. I meet many people who live their lives without passion and drag themselves through their days and nights as if it's a chore. They have lost their dreams and way and seem to be going through the motions of existence with little more to show for it than a few wrinkles and a bad back. Once they see what is possible for their future, they leave their suitcases of beliefs and excuses behind and enter into a new reality where they can raise their vibration and change their destiny. Armed with new tools, they have the potential to be unstoppable, but it is still their choice.

My divining rod is joy, and all decisions I make about everything I do are based on this idea: things either bring me closer to joy or further away. That is the priority that works for me and brings me the most peace. As I continue to do the work for myself and others, this has become a non-negotiable. It attracts other high vibrating people, events, and opportunities from both expected and unexpected sources. Every day is full of inspiring synchronicities, and I am grateful for the divine appointments which fill my calendar. We all have a choice, and I choose joy every time. It always leads me to the miraculous.

THE MEDICINE

Crafting a new mindset around creating an abundant life takes a little work. It is not difficult but does take some practice. I do not focus on the beliefs which need to be replaced because that will attract more things you do not want. Ultimately those outdated ways of thinking get forced out once the new beliefs get a firm hold in your day-to-day actions. You are where you are for a reason, but that doesn't mean you have to stay there.

Prosperity consciousness is not just about money, but it is a good place to start. It is about embracing the idea that there is always more than enough for everyone in all areas from all resources. This flies directly in the face of what most of us are taught from a very young age so this is where we begin.

Start with baby steps to create a transformation that is not overwhelming. We cannot get to the next level until we deal with the truth about where we are right now, and it starts with a decree. You must want change more than you want to stay frozen in time and be willing to speak it out loud. Not-enoughness is our safe place where nothing extra is required, but it is where hopes and dreams go to die if they are left unattended.

Next, you must pay attention to your self-talk. Words are energy that attract results. The universe is always listening, and so is your body and your future. It is up to you to create the happiest, healthiest, most prosperous version of yourself because no one is coming to save you. Your inner and outer conversations create both your inner and outer worlds, so choose each word and phrase wisely. They are seeds for a new reality. You can either be a conscious creator or an unconscious creation, but you cannot be both. Extraordinary times call for extraordinary awareness of your words and thoughts. Your dream life is depending on you so pay very close attention.

There is a reward to struggle, but it is the booby prize. Start dropping quantum currency in your energy bank and buckle your seat belt for a life filled with meaning, passion, and purpose. By cultivating a grateful heart first thing every morning, you will begin to live in a space of gratitude which brings more things to be grateful for every day.

Find your divining rod to act as your rudder. For me, it is joy, and for others, it may be peace, love, freedom, or fame. Let this be the fuel that lights your fire, igniting your God Spark where you become limitless potential.

And finally, say yes to you and invest in yourself with the right tools in your toolbox. Take a giant leap and hire a virtual assistant, a bookkeeper, an organizer, a coach, a housekeeper, a private chef, or a professional muse. Never be afraid to get clear, confident, and courageous. Once you become fearless, you can help others who are still hiding. Giving someone hope guarantees the impossible.

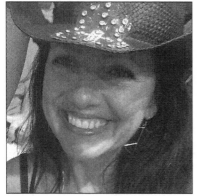

Darlene "The Herbmom" de la Plata has been restoring hope since 1987 by helping clients co-create positive action plans for health and prosperity through Abundant Health & Wealth Services, where financial fitness and optimal well-being are inevitable. This ministry bridges the gap between religion and metaphysics and explores the unconscious roots of dis-ease and lack.

Believing transformation is our birthright, she offers classes, seminars, courses, and coaching programs. This includes the Abundance Academy, a six-week paradigm shift into the world of coherence, prosperity consciousness, wealth strategies, ancestral patterns, and generational curses around success and money.

Her simple healing techniques include education, prayer, light, frequency, specialized supplements, and Seed to Seal premium essential oils. Her motto is "Bring It" because no topic is too tough to tackle. She can help you rise above challenges using tools from the quantum, the physical, and the spiritual realms to help you discover your brilliance.

Allow yourself to step into your divine destiny where infinite possibilities exist. Call today to transcend the limitations of your earthly genealogy and ignite your God spark. You are a Kindred Photon and were born to shine bright. Procrastination can only dim your sparkle and steal your dreams with permission.

Darlene "The Herbmom" de la Plata is an Ordained Minister, Fierce Health Warrior, Visionary Coach, Amazon Explorer, Wealth Strategist, and Professional Muse. She is always in the right place at the right time with all the right people and lives every moment in gratitude. Creating art, experiencing nature, collecting books, and adopting cats are a few of her passions, but her greatest joy is her family. She is a proud YaYa to her grandbabies, who inspire her to be more magical every day and to heal humanity one kindred photon at a time.

www.TheHerbmom.com

404-399-8855

CLOSING CHAPTER

Thank you for exploring SACRED MEDICINE and embracing the wisdom shared by this talented group of authors.

No matter what led you to pick up a copy of this book, you now have 25 sacred medicine teachings to escort you further into self-discovery, healing and to craft your own sacred medicine.

I encourage you to reach out to our team of authors and share your experiences. They offer whole-hearted healing opportunities and are dedicated to making an impact in the lives of others.

They'd love to hear from you, and so would I. Reach out, drop a message, and connect with us on social media or visit our websites.

Walk your path fiercely,

Jen Piceno

If you enjoyed this book, please leave an Amazon review to help share our work on a wider scale. It helps every author in this book share their message with the world and helps readers make purchases that are right for them.

ABOUT JEN PICENO

GET READY TO ALIGN WITH EVERYTHING
YOU WERE MEANT TO BE IN WAYS YOU'VE
NEVER EXPERIENCED BEFORE.

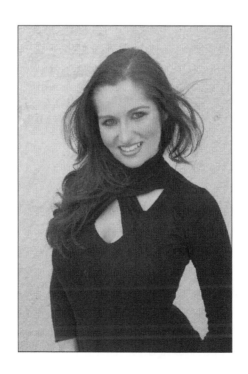

Transform challenging and traumatic life experiences into aligned purpose and step into what you came to this earth to conquer. Jen will teach you how to give self-doubt the middle finger so you can claim your power and walk your path fiercely into your heart's deepest desires.

She's an intuitive life management practitioner, energy medicine specialist, and badass coach with 30+ years of expertise in the healing arts. Through personalized ceremony, generational healing, and channeling the divine, she'll help you bust through restrictions so you can solidify your purpose and begin the transformation you've been craving in all areas of life.

Align with everything you're meant to be in ways you've never experienced before.

We know there are a lot of self-proclaimed priestesses out there, **but Jen is the real deal!** She is an Ordained Shamanic Priestess in the powerful lineage of StarrFire OrbWeaver, Anyaa McAndrew, and the creatrix, Nicole Christine. She walks the priestess path with a level of integrity and purpose as the high priestesses who walked before her. Jen celebrates life in everyday ceremony and is committed to making a radical difference in the lives of others.

She leads women through some of life's toughest challenges.

As a ceremonialist, her programs offer one-of-a-kind, personalized sacred experiences that **shatter old beliefs and empower unlimited abundance in all areas of life.**

She activates, aligns, and attunes women with their highest potential – women are seen, heard, and appreciated like never before. Check out the social proof and reviews – She's transforming lives!

Are you ready for this?

When you say "yes" to the experience, she'll take you on a magical adventure – it's the best part!

Working in sacredness and manifesting desires unified with our highest potential makes a massive difference in how women show up in life and how people see and value their worth.

Jen believes that everyone has the potential to make an impact in the lives of others. She believes that everyone is a change-maker.

Unfortunately, most people are unintentionally creating what they don't want. No worries, she'll take care of that!

Jen will guide you through practices that easily integrate with contemporary lives to support your heart's deepest desires so you can walk your path fiercely with confidence to get what you want most.

She is a gifted ceremonialist, cacao practitioner, and culinary enthusiast. She weaves food, dance, culture, and diversity into her work to create sacred experiences that awaken all the senses and share teachings of intentional living in delicious ways.

Jen is a Reiki Master directly attuned in all levels by the world-renowned Reiki Master Diane Stein, author of Essential Reiki. Those who receive Reiki training from Jen receive this powerful lineage. Jen's also trained in Energy Balancing and karmic release with Diane Stein.

Jen's fertility battle taught her all about the power found in womb work and ceremonial healings. She lived in Mexico for two months and traveled there yearly for over a decade. She was ignited and brought into this work by several different elders along the way.

She worked with expert curanderas, sobadoras, and shamans. She was initiated all over Mexico in private homes and sacred sites. She studied Mayan abdominal massage, Toltec wisdom, and shamanism with spiritual leaders and elders here in the US.

Jen is a Womb Keeper initiated in a lineage of women through jungle medicine. She carries the 13th rite of the Munay-Ki: Rite of the Womb, along with the original nine rites held in sacredness to pass to those seeking to connect to divine luminous beings through this lineage.

Jen shares these sacred gifts with spiritually mature women rooted in integrity to make the world a better place.

HER EMPIRE:

Jen is building an empire where women can finally exit survival mode and step into ecstatic living. They're drawn into liberation with a rush of adrenaline. Saying "yes" to yourself does that!

It allows women to thrive. It feels so damn good and comes in full throttle when women wake up and remember who they are. They finally give self-doubt the middle finger so they can live the life their heart desires.

What a rush that is! They're more alive, energetic, and confident – they glow with magnificence and start getting the attention they deserve.

Enter this kingdom with Jen as your guide. She'll take you on a journey to exactly who you are called to be. That's much different than who you were conditioned or told to be. Round up the courage to step through the door, and she will lift you up and teach you how to be an unstoppable force of nature.

She's a mysterious magical being, and this place is completely enchanted. You're protected. It's safe to be honest, outspoken, playful, and free-spirited. It's encouraged here! Isn't it time to be with someone that's got your back? She'll ignite your power and invite it to stay awhile so you can discover the essence of who you are.

HER COMPANY – GYPSY MOON, INC.

As a truth-seeker and lifetime student of the healing arts, Jen is the CEO of Gypsy Moon Inc. She's a master of the creative healing arts teaching ecstatic life management, self-mastery, personal and spiritual development, and wealth consciousness.

Her programs and retreats encourage women to develop intuitive abilities and learn new techniques to expand so they can heal the past, align with purpose, and step into their divine powers with confidence.

https://JenPiceno.com

WHAT PEOPLE ARE SAYING:

"Truly a Woman's Woman! Jen's passion for knowledge, attention to detail, and dedication to helping others is such an inspiration as she fearlessly contributes her gifts to the world. She is a beautiful person, and her energy is just amazing!"

~Bronwyn

"I love Jen Piceno! Jen is an amazing teacher and ceremonialist. She uses body, mind, spirit, and creativity to help you move through blocks and embrace your authentic self. Her sessions help heal the past and connect you to your heart again!"

~Sarah Friday

"I honestly didn't know what I was getting into when I met this tiny powerhouse. She is fierce and beautiful and larger than life. And her work…well, it is nothing short of magical!"

~Bridget Maddocks

"I have had the honor of being a part of what Jen Piceno is doing for the last several months. Jen has a way of getting to the truth of a matter in minutes. She has an innate ability to see what's going on and be available for the solution. She doesn't play small and doesn't allow you to either. I have grown more in the last few months of working with her than I have in almost a decade of personal growth work. I cannot recommend her enough."

~Erin Jones, Urban Evolution Salon

Jen is full of fire and passion that she pours out to others. She loves what she does, and it shows whether she is healing or teaching. I have experienced Jen in both contexts, and at all times, she is fully present to steer you through your muck. I am always impressed with the questions she asks to enlighten you. I always experience a "lightbulb" moment working with her. No matter how much you're drowning in darkness, Jen will gently guide you to feeling lighter and brighter! But the best part of Jen is her infectious humor. She makes the world a better place.

~Debbie Marshall

"Jen has the ability to deeply connect to Spirit and hold space for the gifts and blessings of each individual. She's an authentic heart-centered leader."

~Lisa Michaels, Author of *Natural Rhythms:*
A Sacred Guide Into Nature's Creation Secrets

"Jen is a caring, compassionate and fierce healing soul with knowledge and magic to share with everyone who comes to her."

~Emily Francis, Author of *The Body Heals Itself*

"When I first asked Jen to lead a session with the co-authors of my book *Find Your Voice, Save Your Life*, my thought was simply about offering a session on celebrating having written our stories for the book. Honestly, I didn't know exactly what to expect. In her most powerful way, Jen took us from a place of acknowledging our work and seeing our words as our own power to help other women heal to a place of being embraced by our ancestral grandmothers, supporting us to do more. Thanks to Jen, we are off on a challenge to celebrate ourselves, not just today but each day coming. Jen is a spiritual powerhouse who can work with you personally but also create an incredibly impactful session for your groups or your clients."

~Dianna Leeder, Crave More Life Coaching,
and author of *Find Your Voice, Save Your Life*

AN ABUNDANCE
OF GRATITUDE

Living life ecstatically, consciously, and abundantly is found easily in a state of gratitude. Within the frequency of gratitude, we become magnetic forces for attracting desires into our life experience with ease and grace.

This powerful truth anchors us more deeply into consciousness and invites abundance to flow into all areas of life. It welcomes in riches without us chasing after it.

Within this frequency, I send deep gratitude to our authors, the medicine men and women who shared their stories, expertise, and sacred medicine. Thank you for making beautiful magic together as brothers and sisters for this mystical collaboration. Thank you for trusting me to lead this project and for coming together on this writing adventure side by side in unity. Together we're already changing lives.

To my husband and son, thank you for the gift of love and laughter that fills our home day and night and all the perfectly imperfect space in between. I learn, stretch, and grow with all the experiences we share.

To our readers, thank you for being here with an open heart, ready to receive what we so dearly hold sacred. As you anchor into the magic and mystery through this transformational medicine, know you are loved and deeply appreciated today and always. The sacred medicine we offer you throughout this book is a resource to guide you on your journey. Return to its pages as needed and soak up its wisdom. May you attract an abundance of love, health, happiness, and wealth into your life along the way and share it with others on their journey.

To our book designer, Dino Marino, thank you for making this book extra magical.

To our cover artist, Diana Toma, thank you for gracing our cover with your gorgeous art. It is divine!

To all of our family, friends, colleagues, and book launch team members, thank you for your support throughout the duration of this project. We couldn't have done it without you.

To my dear friend Lulu Trevena, thank you for trusting your intuition and leading me onto the writer's journey. I'm an author because of you. Thank you for being on this adventure with me.

To Pat Perrier, thank you for your support and all the wisdom you shared to help me become a better writer with my first three books. You gave me the courage to keep writing.

To Amy Gillespie Dougherty, thank you for inviting me to write for The Ancestors Within; it was an experience that opened me up and led me to write this book.

Big love and so much gratitude to Laura Di Franco and Brave Healer Productions. Thank you for your badass coaching, incredible support, and for encouraging us all to share our brave words with the world one book at a time.

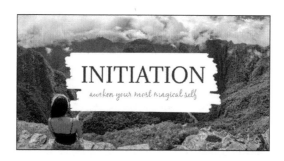

CIRCLE UP FOR A MAGICAL 8-WEEK ONLINE GROUP COACHING EXPERIENCE

- The Elements – Earth wisdom and everyday magic
- Develop intuition, psychic gifts, and self-healing practices.
- The art of ceremony and the power of creating sacred space.
- Introduction to deeper healing: release fears and get honest self-reflection with shadow work.
- Work with your energetic body and learn self-help techniques.

COURSE OVERVIEW
INTERACTIVE GROUP LEARNING EXPERIENCE:

- Meet every two weeks with time to integrate practices in-between live (or Zoom) meetings
- Access to 2 master instructors for deep support
- Detailed instructions for ceremonies that you can use whenever you like.
- Access to a private FB group to support you on your journey.

Bonus:

Each meeting includes potent energetics to accelerate your personal healing experience.

- Receive activations for each element (earth, water, air, fire) for deeper healing.
- Plus, group light body activations to awaken your most magical self

Learn More Here: https://www.JenPiceno.com

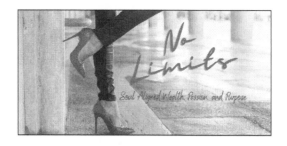

WEALTH CONSCIOUSNESS COACHING & SOUL ALIGNED LIFE MANAGEMENT

WITH JEN PICENO

Customized private programs to transform all areas of life.

You'll get therapeutic healing, integrative spiritual practices, and badass intuitive coaching rolled into one. It'll take you on a mighty adventure into wealth consciousness and soul-aligned life management!

Get ready to:

- Bust through blocks like you never thought possible.
- Transform emotional chaos, mental fatigue, and physical exhaustion into personal power.
- Experience a magical connection that blasts through self-doubt and enhances all areas of life.
- Get information and strategies for yourself and your business other coaches cannot provide.
- Learn how to trust your gut and lean into intuition.
- Quickly get to the heart of your deepest desires with a clear path forward.
- Simplify life.
- Live a beautifully integrated ecstatic life doing what you love.

Journey with me, your wealth consciousness coach, transformation teacher, priestess, and guide, on a path of limitless possibilities.

Finally, understand what's in the way of the magical life you know is waiting for you.

Learn about the spiritual/psychic gifts and sacred purpose you were put on earth to experience and raise your vibration to step into wealth consciousness (relationships, health, finances, happiness, love, and business).

Through multi-sensory experiences, including ancestral healing and energetic clearings, you'll move from fatigue and scarcity into abundance in all areas of life.

Receive channeled messages from the divine that helps heal past wounds, lift pain, and bring profound clarity faster than standard coaching.

We'll get you where you've been longing to go!

https://JenPiceno.com

HIRE TO JEN TO SPEAK AT YOUR NEXT EVENT

Book Jen Piceno for podcast interviews, special appearances, and retreats that center around any of the following themes:

- Health and wellness
- Women's empowerment
- Personal development
- Spiritual growth
- The art of ceremony
- Energy medicine
- Embodiment and integration
- Mindset
- Wealth consciousness

Contact Jen at https://www.JenPiceno.com

JOIN THE AUTHOR TEAM FOR JEN'S NEXT COLLABORATIVE BOOK

Join me; I'm collaborating with teachers, magic-makers, healers, mystics, and experts in their field of study who are ready to share their message with the world in a bigger way!

Contributing a chapter to these meaningful collaborative projects is much more than having your name on a book cover.

It's about being part of a community of expert practitioners and entrepreneurs who are changing the world with their brave words, wisdom, experience, and heart-centered healing practices.

Each author shares a personal story and teaches an effecting self-healing practice in their chapter. Authors then have opportunities to do live training, podcast interviews, and business development activities as a part of the Brave Healer Productions family.

I can't wait to hear your story!

To explore opportunities for my next book project, please reach out to schedule a chat by emailing fierce@JenPiceno.com

OTHER BOOKS
WITH JEN PICENO:

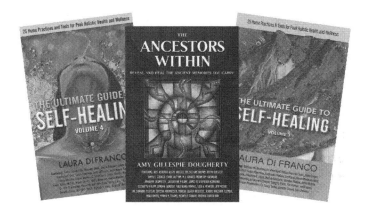

The Ultimate Guide to Self-Healing, Volume 3
Chapter 16
Energetic Womb Healing:
Reclaiming Your Feminine Power and Fertility Naturally

The Ultimate Guide to Self-Healing, Volume 4
Chapter 3
Balancing Codependence:
Finding Self-Acceptance and Personal Power

The Ancestors Within,
Reveal and Heal the Ancient Memories You Carry
Chapter 23
Ancestral Power:
Claim Your Sacred Wisdom and Magic

Purchase signed copies here: https://www.JenPiceno.com/books

CEREMONIAL GRADE CACAO

TO ENHANCE SPIRITUAL AND MAGICAL EXPERIENCES

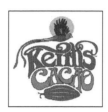

Jen Piceno is a registered Cacao Practitioner with Keith's Cacao – Ceremonial Grade Guatemalan Cacao from the Chocolate Shaman.

This powerful superfood is a delicious plant medicine with many benefits and uses:

- Consciousness & Spirituality
- Workplace Productivity
- Creativity and Art
- Athletics and Physical Training
- Healthy Living
- Heart-Opening Awareness

**BUY NOW - Get your Cacao here with my affiliate discount link:
http://www.keithscacao.com/discount/piceno18us62**

DELICIOUS CACAO RESOURCES:

- Basic Ceremonial Cacao Recipe: http://www.jenpiceno.com/resources
- Jen's Aphrodite Ritual with Sacred Cacao:
  https://jenpiceno.com/aphrodite-cacao-ritual/

Thank you for delving into the pages of this book. I'll leave you with this ancient shamanic blessing translated from Nahuatl.

May the beauty of each release serve you well.

Big Love,

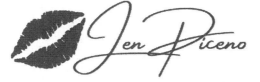

I RELEASE

"I release my partner from the obligation to complete me.

I release my parents from the feeling they failed with me.

I release my children from the need to bring me pride, so they can write their own paths to the rhythm of their hearts as it whispers in their ear.

I don't lack anything; I learn from all beings, all the time.

Thanking my grandparents and ancestors who came together to allow me to be alive and follow my path today.

I release them from past failures and unfulfilled desires, knowing they have done their best to travel their way of living with their standard of consciousness.

I strip my soul before their eyes;
that's why they know I don't hide or owe anything.

I must be faithful to myself more than ever by walking with heart
wisdom. I know that I am fulfilling my life project,
free from family loyalties that can disrupt my peace and happiness.
This detachment is my responsibility.

I surrender the role of the savior to be the one who unites or meets
the expectations of others.

I cherish my essence, my way of expressing it, e
ven if not everyone can understand me.

I honor you; I love you and recognize your innocence.

I honor the divinity in me and you...

We are free."

_____